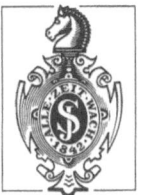

Kinya Ishikawa

Adnexal Tumors of the Skin

An Atlas

With 116 Figures

Springer-Verlag
Tokyo Berlin Heidelberg New York
London Paris

Dr. KINYA ISHIKAWA

Department of Dermatology
Kasumigaura National Hospital
7-14, Shimotakatsu 2-chome
Tsuchiura, 300 Japan

Library of Congress Cataloging-in-Publication Data
Ishikawa, Kinya, 1923–
Adnexal tumors of the skin.
Includes bibliographies and index. 1. Skin—Tumors—Atlases. 2. Hair follicles
—Tumors—Atlases. 3. Sweat glands—Tumors—Atlases. I. Title. [DNLM:
1. Skin Appendage Diseases—pathology—atlases. 2. Skin Neoplasms—pathology
—atlases. 3. Sweat Gland Neoplasms—pathology—atlases. WR 17 I79a]
RC280.S5I84   1987   616.99′2770758   87-4603
ISBN-13: 978-4-431-68056-7   e-ISBN-13: 978-4-431-68054-3
DOI: 10.1007/ 978-4-431-68054-3

This work is subject to copyright. All rights are reserved, whether the whole or part
of the material is concerned, specifically the rights of translation, reprinting, reuse
of illustrations, recitation, broadcasting, reproduction on microfilms or in other
ways, and storage in data banks.

© Springer-Verlag Tokyo 1987
Softcover reprint of the hardcover 1st edition 1987

The use of registered names, trademarks, etc. in this publication does not imply, even
in the absence of a specific statement, that such names are exempt from the relevant
protective laws and regulations and therefore free for general use.

Product liability: The publisher can give no guarantee for information about drug
dosage and application thereof contained in this book. In every individual case
the respective user must check its accuracy by consulting other pharmaceutical
literature.

Typesetting: Asco Trade Typesetting Ltd., Hong Kong

Preface

Toward a full understanding of the skin adrexa and associated tumors, an accurate and detailed visual record of the various structures encountered is essential. Such a comprehensive survey has, however, hitherto been lacking in works on dermatology; this situation I attempt to remedy in the present atlas by presenting a collection of my own cases over the years. I took almost all the photomicrographs myself using a Nikon Biophot microscope.

I would like to express my deep gratitude to Prof. Hitoshi Hatano, Department of Dermatology, School of Medicine, Keio University, who reviewed this book and consented to its publication. I am especially grateful to Dr. Junya Fukuda, Chief Pathologist, Kawasaki Municipal Hospital, who helped in diagnosing routine histological sections of the skin and gave invaluable advice with this book. I am enormously indebted to Mr. Soichi Narutomi, Chief Technician, Section of Pathology, Kawasaki Municipal Hospital, who produced first-class prints from 35-mm films. I must express my deep thanks to the late Mr. Shin Takeichi, Head of Photography, Department of Pathology, School of Medicine, Keio University, who kindly took photomicrographs for me for many years; some of these are included in the present volume. I owe a great deal to Associate Prof. Kan Niizuma, Department of Dermatology, School of Medicine, Tokai University, who kindly arranged for this book to be published by Springer-Verlag. Finally, I should like to acknowledge the efforts and goodwill of Springer-Verlag Tokyo.

Spring, 1987   KINYA ISHIKAWA

Contents

Structure of the Adnexa

HAIR FOLLICLE

Normal structure

REFERENCES

1 Pinkus H (1967) Pathobiology of the pilary complex. Jpn J Dermatol Ser B 77: 304–330
2 Pinkus H (1968) Static and dynamic histology and histochemistry of hair growth. In: Baccaredda-Boy A, Moretti G, Frey JR (eds) Biopathology of pattern alopecia. Karger, Basel, pp 69–81
3 Pinkus H (1978) Epithelial-mesodermal interaction in normal hair growth, alopecia, and neoplasia. J Dermatol (Tokyo) 5: 93–101

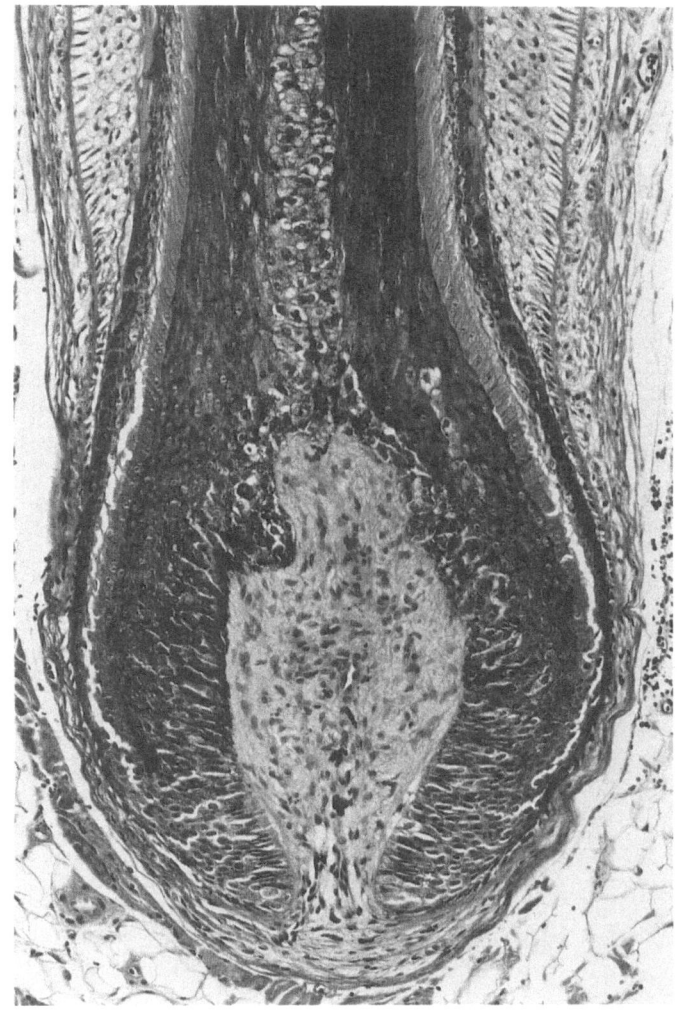

Fig. 1. Matrix area of an anagen hair follicle. The fibrous root sheath protrudes into the bell-shaped hair bulb and forms the dermal papilla, in which papilla cells are seen to be crowded. The specific differentiation of the matrix cells, which is shown in the following figures, is determined by the dermal papilla; it is especially influenced by the linear distance of the cells from the base of the papilla [1–3].
H and E, × 160

Figures 2–15 are photomicrographs of a huge hair follicle found in a section of intradermal nevus on the neck of a 26-year-old man. Because the hair follicle is somewhat obliquely sectioned, all of the dermal papilla is confined within the hair bulb.

Fig. 2. The hair matrix portion. Six kinds of pilar keratinocyte are differentiating from the outside to the ▷ inside of the hair matrix: (1) Henle's layer (*He*), (2) Huxley's layer (*Hu*), (3) cuticle of the inner root sheath (*CI*), (4) cuticle of the hair (*CH*), (5) hair cortex (*Co*), and (6) hair medulla (*M*). Lateral to these, three sheaths are seen: (1) outer root sheath (*ORS*), (2) vitreous (or glassy) membrane (*VM*), and (3) fibrous root sheath (*FRS*).
H and E, × 500

FRS VM ORS He Hu Cl CH Co M

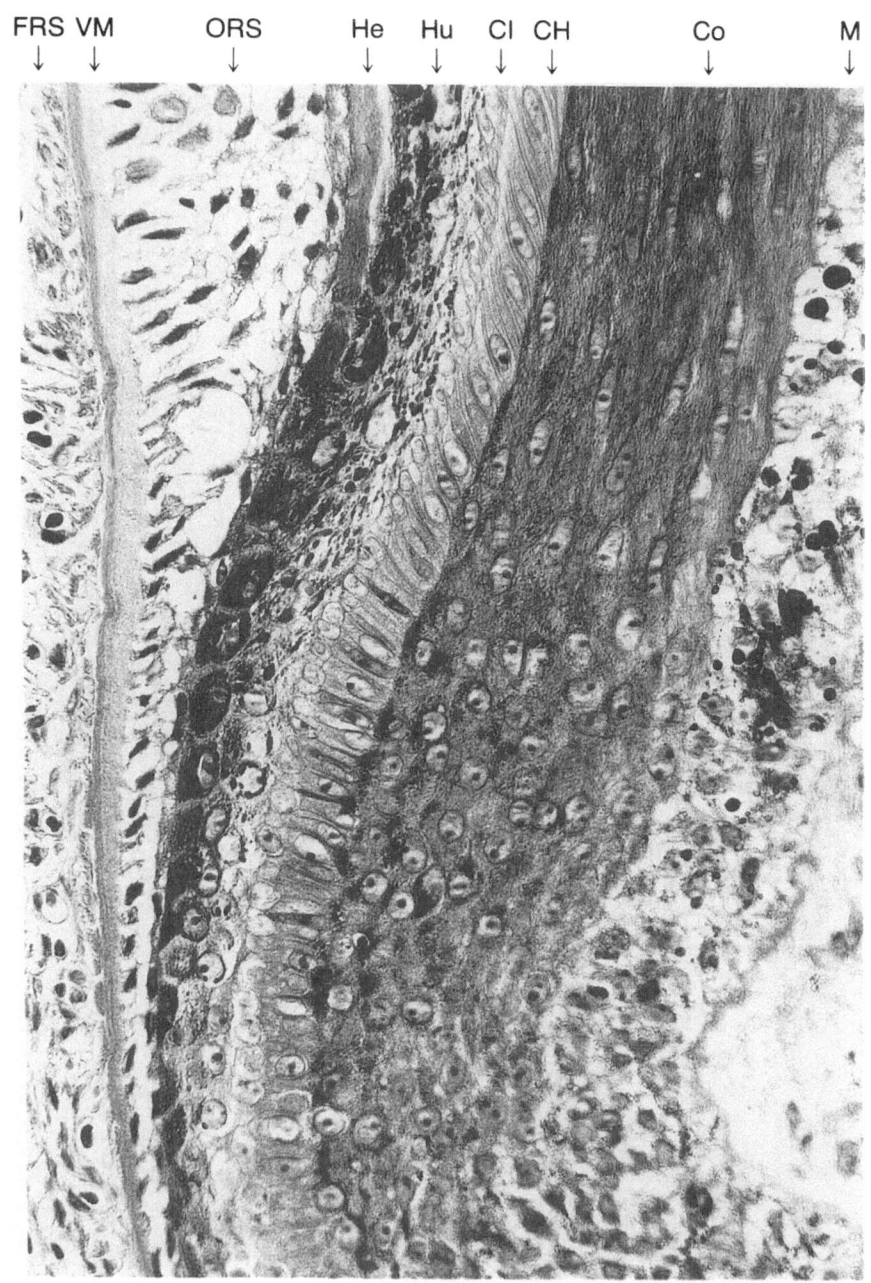

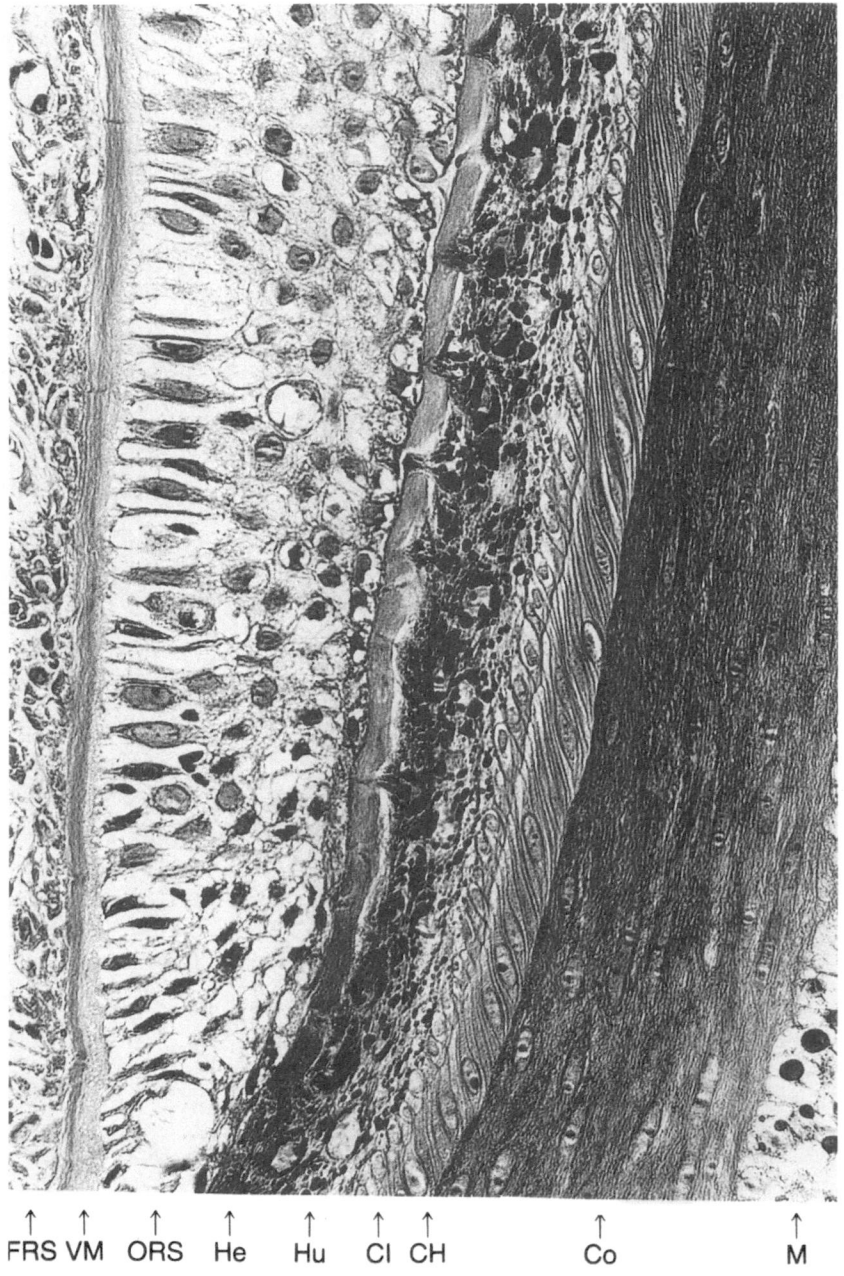

FRS VM ORS He Hu CI CH Co M

Fig. 3. A somewhat higher portion. Figures 2 and 3 partly overlap.
H and E, × 500

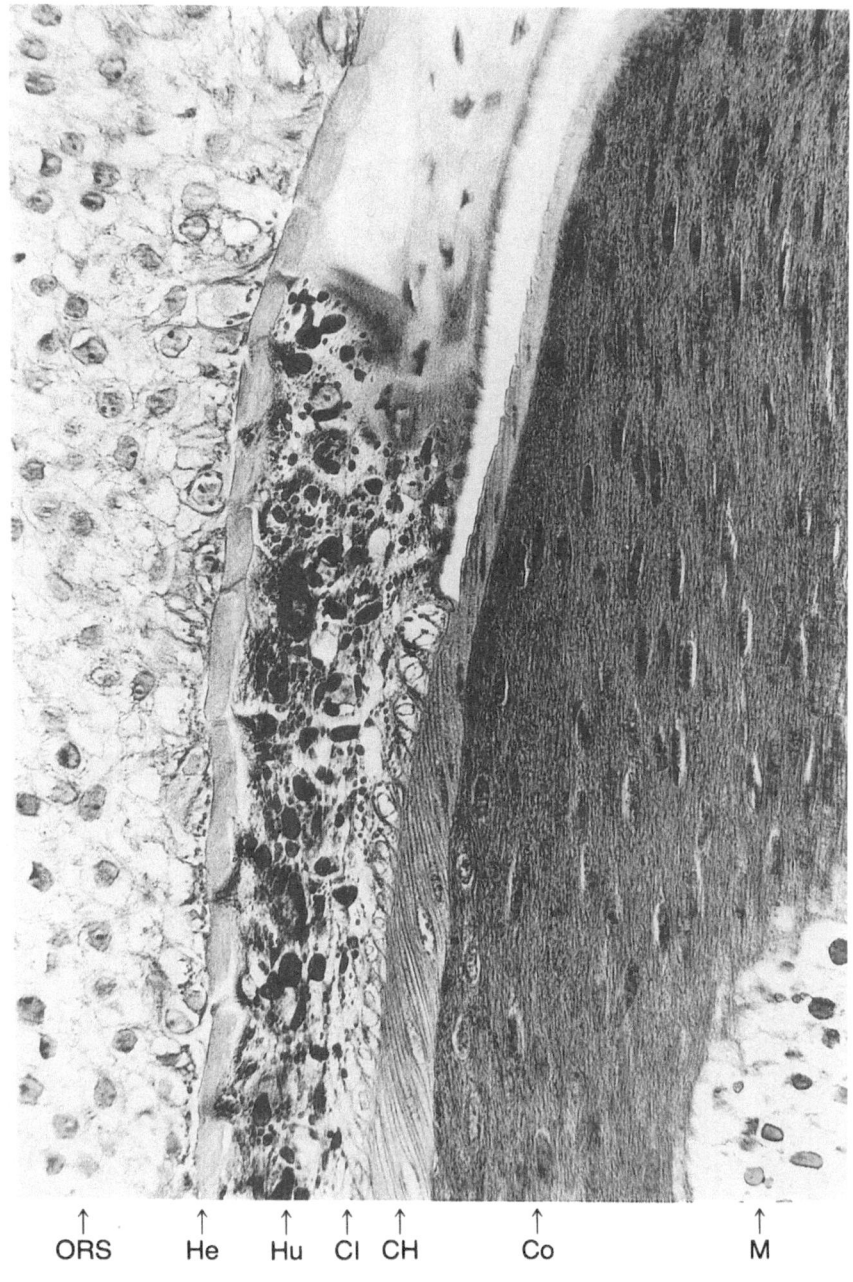

Fig. 4. A still higher portion than Fig. 3. Figures 3 and 4 partly overlap.
H and E, × 500

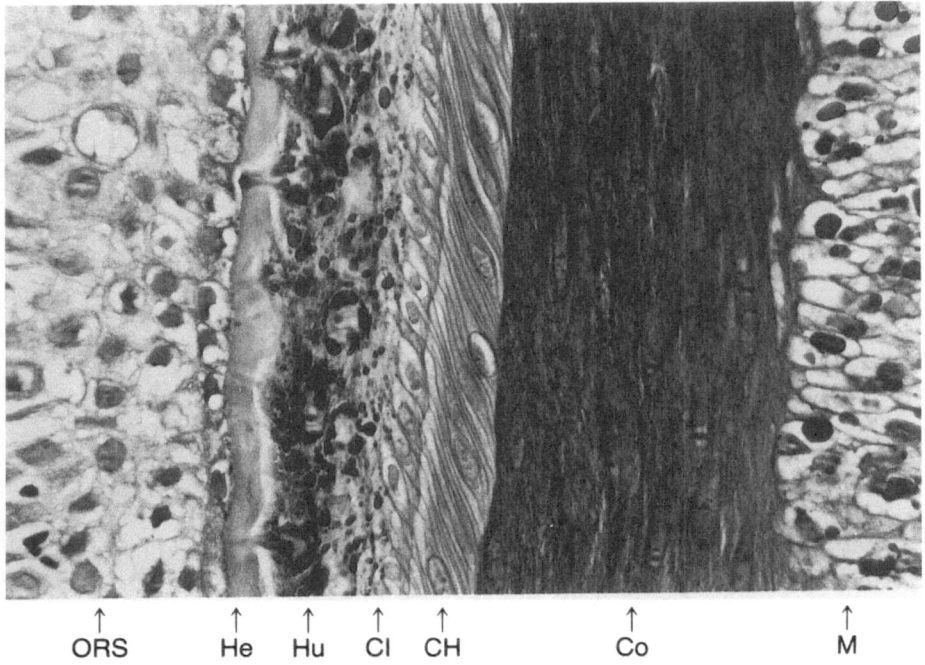

ORS He Hu Cl CH Co M

Fig. 5. Higher magnification of Fig. 3. Different cell groups are shown in detail. At this level, tricho-hyaline granules are seen only in the cells of Huxley's layer and of the medulla.
H and E, × 640

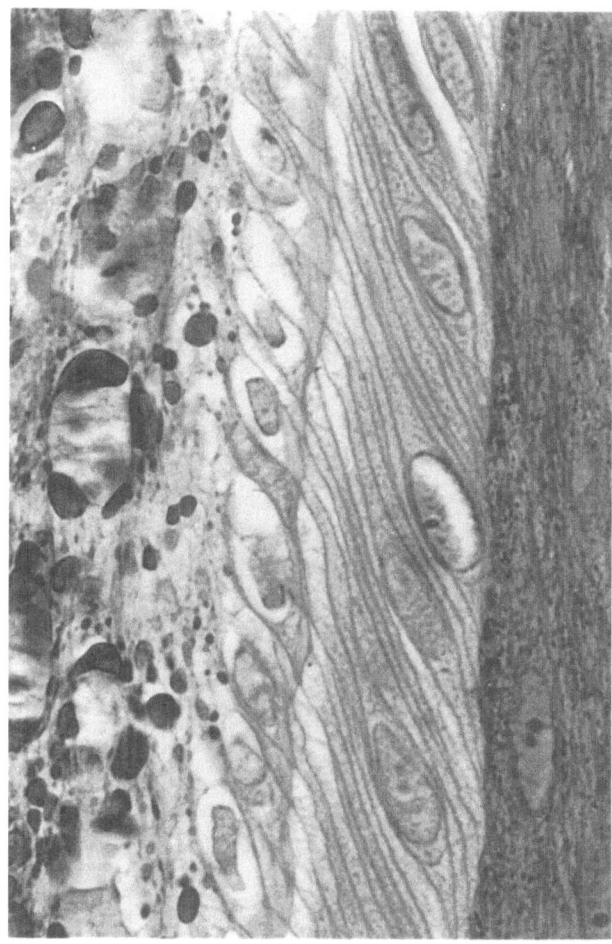

Fig. 6. High magnification of Fig. 5. The cells of the cuticle of the hair tightly interlock with those of the cuticle of the inner root sheath.
H and E, × 1600

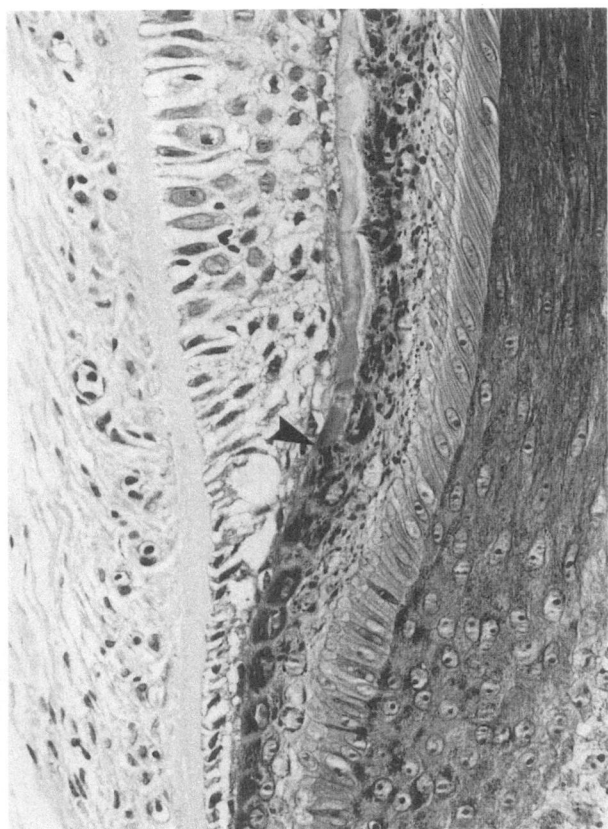

Fig 7. Keratinization of the cells of Henle's layer. The cells of Henle's layer keratinize first. The cells filled with fine trichohyaline granules are abruptly changing into a fully keratinized layer (*arrow*).
H and E, × 400

Fig. 8. Trıchohyalıne granules in the hair medulla. In
the medulla, trichohyaline
granules are seen as large
eosinophılic droplets.
H and E, × 800

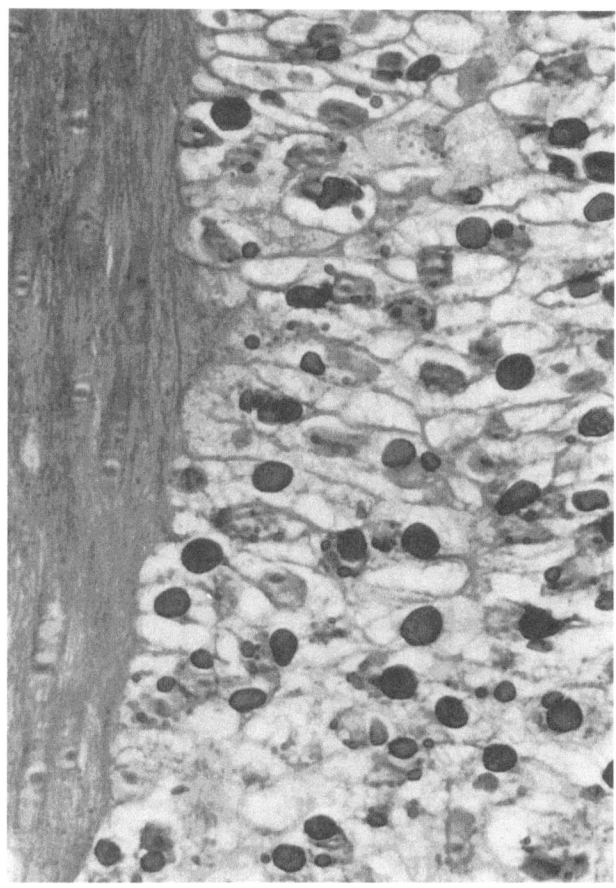

Figures 9–12 show details of the cuticle of the hair and of the inner root sheath at different levels.

Fig. 9. The cells of the cuticle of the hair, after having differentiated from the matrix, become columnar, ▷
directing their long axes at right angles to the axis of the hair.
H and E, × 1600

Fig. 10. The cells then begin gradually to point their outer edges upward.   ▷
H and E, × 1600

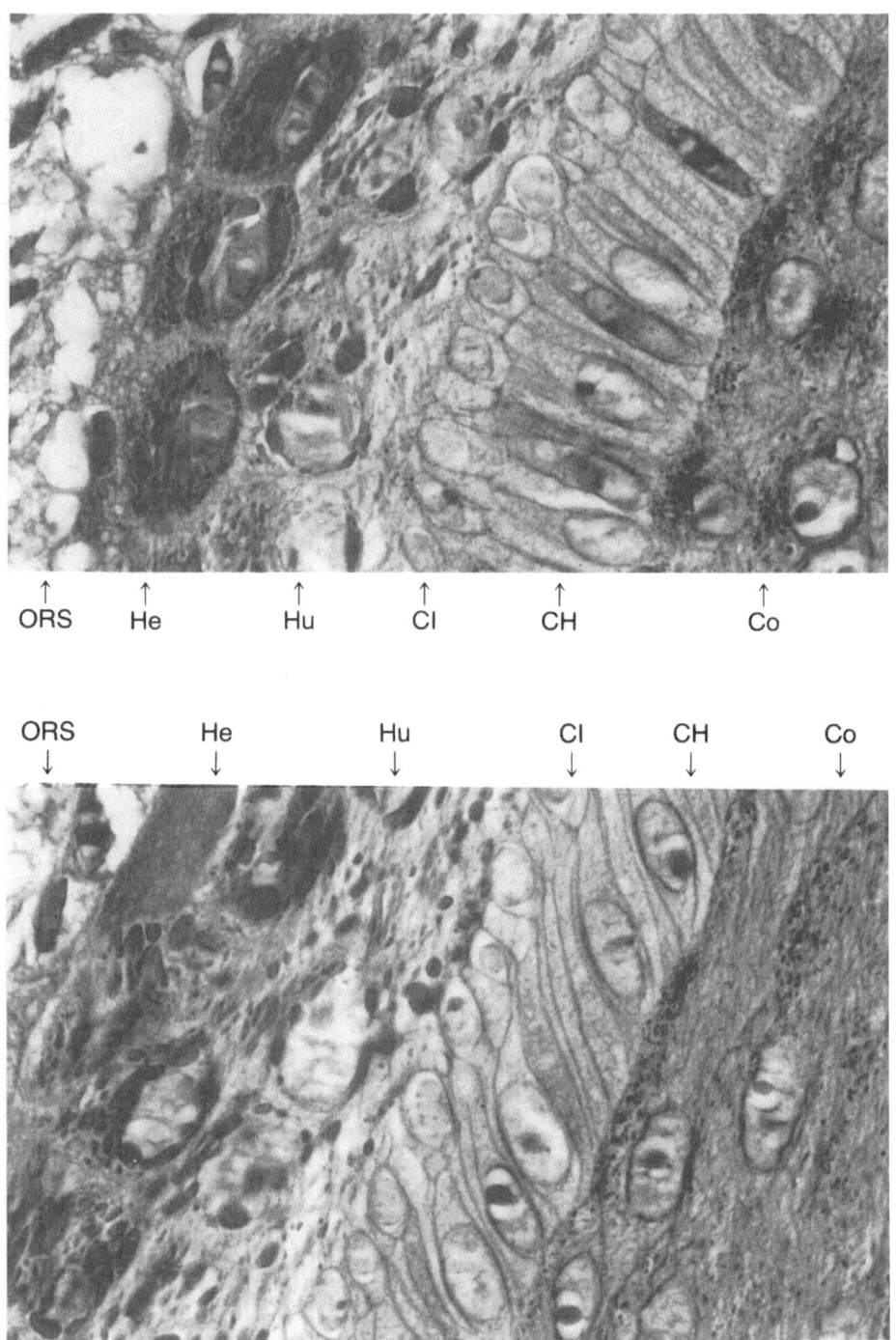

ORS He Hu Cl CH Co

ORS He Hu Cl CH Co

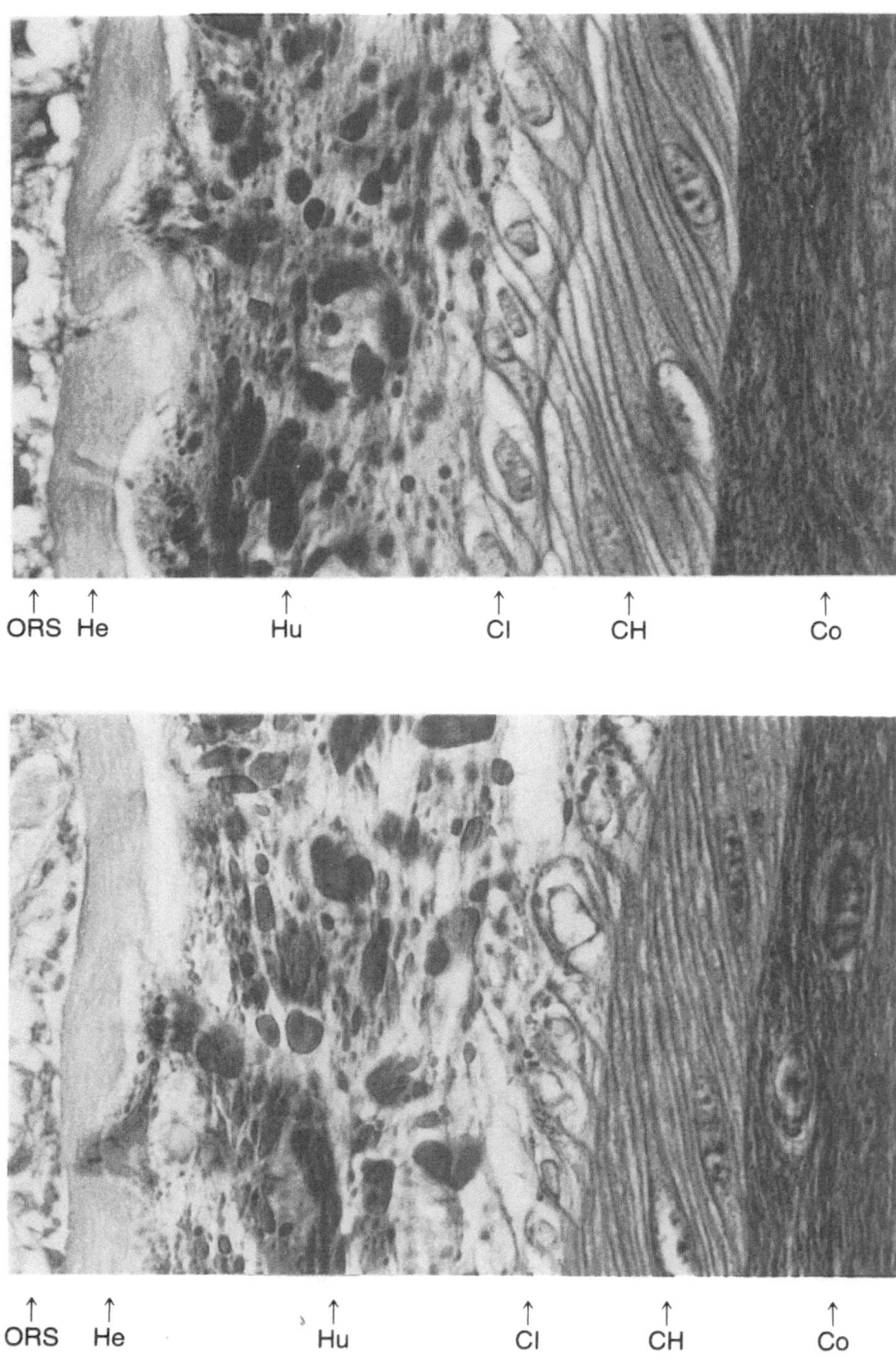

↑   ↑   ↑   ↑   ↑   ↑
ORS   He   Hu   Cl   CH   Co

↑   ↑   ↑   ↑   ↑   ↑
ORS   He   Hu   Cl   CH   Co

Fig. 13. Fully keratinized cuticle of the hair (*right*) and inner root sheath (*left*). Both are free of interlocking.
H and E, × 2000

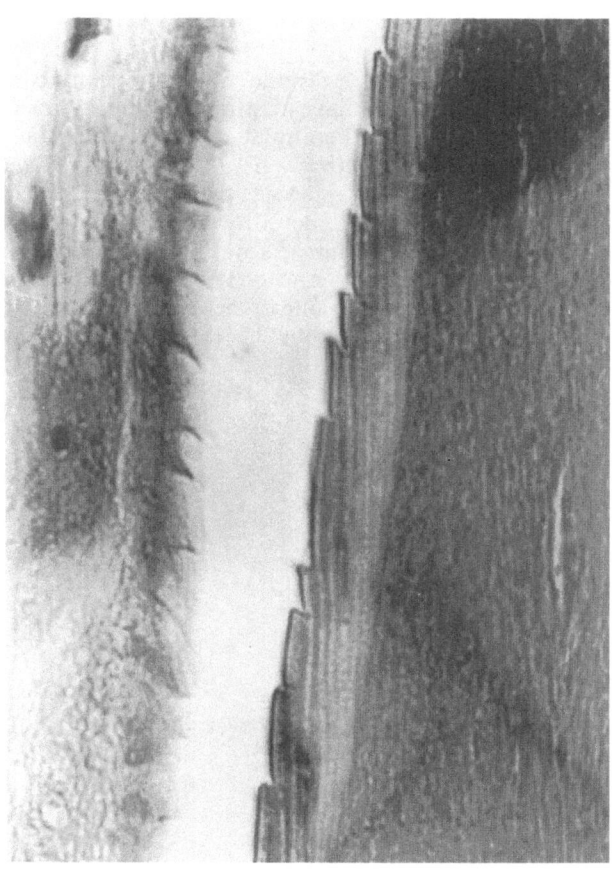

REFERENCES

1 Lever WF, Schaumburg-Lever G (1983) Histopathology of the skin, 6th edn. Lippincott, Philadelphia, pp 25–29
2 Montagna W (1962) The structure and function of skin, 2nd edn. Academic Press, New York, pp 181–200
3 Pinkus H, Mehregan AH (1981) A guide to dermatohistopathology, 3rd edn. Appleton-Century-Crofts, New York, pp 25–28

◁ *Fig. 11.* The cells grow more and more flattened and become obliquely arranged, thin, overlapping cells. The cells of the cuticle of the inner root sheath are at first cuboidal and arranged in contact with the outer edges of the cuticle cells of the hair (Fig. 9). They then become gradually elongated and point their long axes downward (Fig. 10); thus, they begin to interlock tightly with the cuticle cells of the hair (Fig. 11).
H and E, × 1600

◁ *Fig. 12.* At a high level, trichohyaline granules are seen appearing in the cuticle cells of the inner root sheath.
H and E, × 1600

15

Flügelzellen (Hoepke)

In the fully keratinized Henle's layer, openings can be observed at intervals. After the live Henle's cells have keratinized, Henle's layer is stretched. Consequently, it is now not a compact keratin sheath but has become a perforated, wickerworklike cylinder (*fischreusenartiges Gebilde*—structure like a fish trap) [6, 7], the meshes of which histologically appear as the openings. Already in the living stage of Henle's cells, some cells of Huxley's layer (*Flügelzellen*) send their cytoplasmic processes (*Flügelfortsätze*) out into the outer root sheath through the intercellular spaces of Henle's layer, and even after keratinization of Henle's layer the processes pass through the above openings. The *Flügelzellen* are regarded as bridges, across which nutrients of the outer root sheath are carried into the still living cells of Huxley's layer [1, 4, 5, 8].

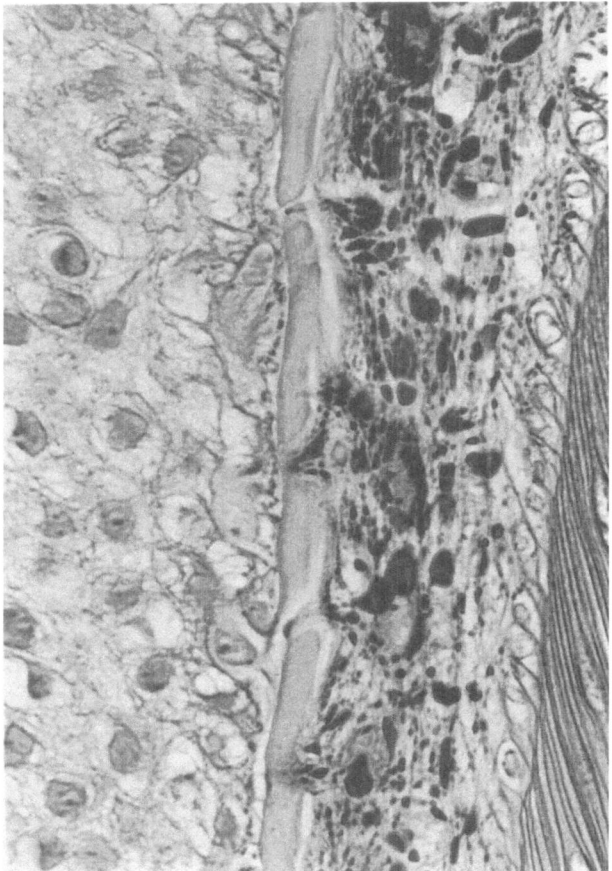

Fig. 14. Openings in Henle's layer through which *Flügelzellen* send out their processes. H and E, × 800

16

Fig. 15. Trichohyaline granules are seen in the processes. Fine trichohyaline granules are also noted flowing between Henle's layer and the outer root sheath.
H and E, × 2000

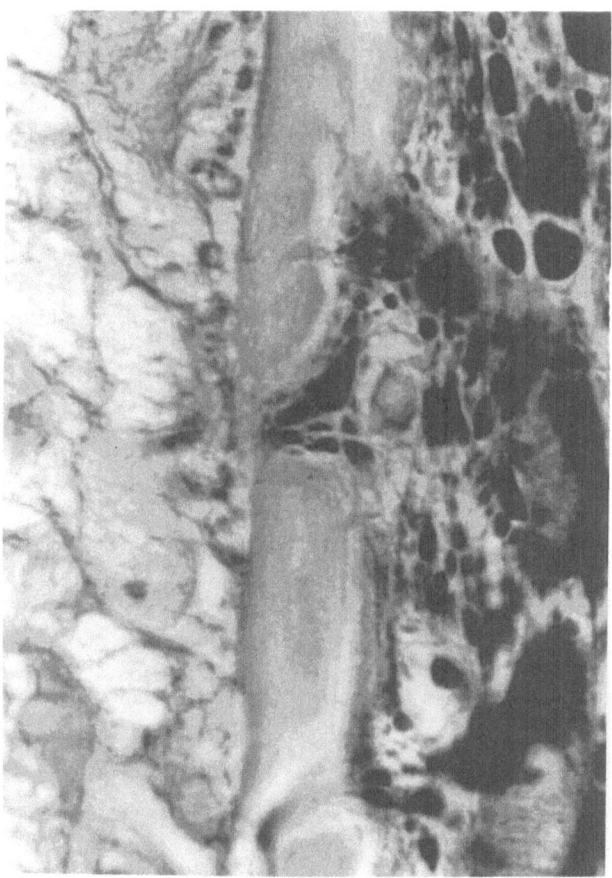

REFERENCES

1 Breathnach AS (1971) An atlas of the ultrastructure of human skin: Development, differentiation, and post-natal features. Churchill, London, pp 294–295, 304–305
2 Happey F, Johnson AG (1962) Some electron microscope observations on hardening in the human hair follicle. J Ultrastruct Res 7: 316–327
3 Hoepke H (1927) Die Haare. In: von Möllendorff W (ed) Handbuch der mikroskopischen Anatomie des Menschen, vol. 3, part 1. Springer, Berlin, pp 74–77
4 Montagna W, Van Scott EJ (1958) The anatomy of the hair follicle. In: Montagna W, Ellis RA (eds) The biology of hair growth. Academic Press, New York, pp 56–57
5 Montagna W (1962) The structure and function of skin, 2nd edn. Academic Press, New York, p 192
6 Pinkus F (1927) Die normale Anatomie der Haut. In: Jadassohn J (ed) Handbuch der Haut- und Geschlechtskrankheiten, vol. 1, part 1. Springer, Berlin, pp 122–125, 200–203
7 Pinkus H (1958) Embryology of hair. In: Montagna W, Ellis RA (eds) The biology of hair growth. Academic Press, New York, p 22
8 Zaun H (1968) Histologie, Histochemie und Wachstumsdynamik des Haarfollikels. In: Marchionini A (ed) Handbuch der Haut- und Geschlechtskrankheiten, Ergänzungswerk, vol. 1, part 1. Springer, Berlin, p 151

Keratogenous zone of hair

The keratogenous zone of hair is the part analogous to the granular cell layer of the epidermis [4]. In this zone, the living cells of the hair cortex change gradually into hard keratin. Trichohyaline granules are found electron microscopically [1]. In fungal disease, an inverted V-shaped Adamson's fringe appears at the upper level of the keratogenous zone because keratinophilic fungi propagate only in mature keratin [2, 5].

REFERENCES

1 Ito M, Hashimoto K (1982) Trichohyaline granules in hair cortex. J Invest Dermatol 79: 392–398
2 Kligman AM (1955) Tinea capitis due to *M. audouini* and *M. canis*: II. Dynamics of the host-parasite relationship. Arch Dermatol 71: 313–337
3 Leblond CP (1951) Histological structure of hair, with a brief comparison to other epidermal appendages and epidermis itself. Ann NY Acad Sci 53: 464–475
4 Lever WF, Schaumburg-Lever G (1983) Histopathology of the skin, 6th edn. Lippincott, Philadelphia, p 11
5 MacKie RM (1984) Milne's dermatopathology. Arnold, London, p 27

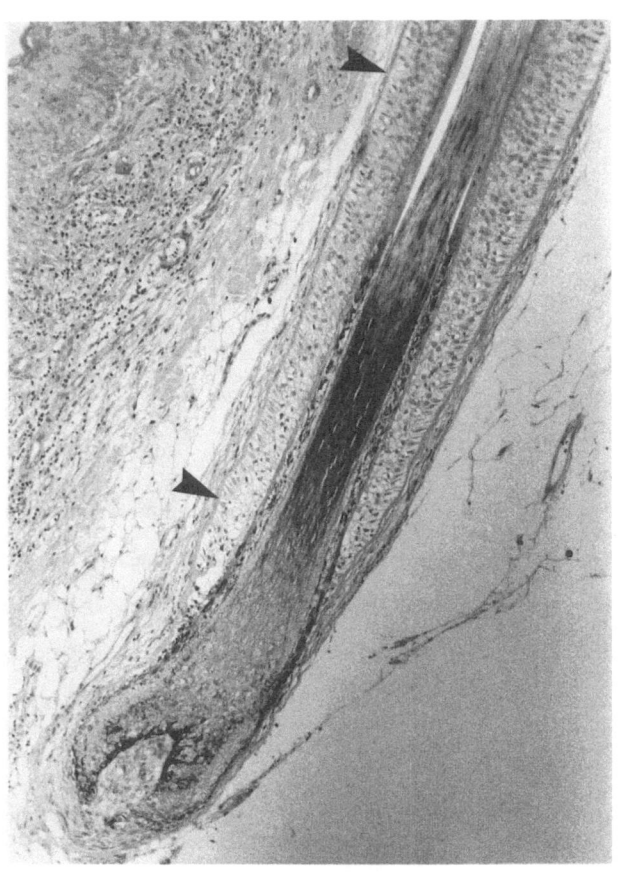

Fig. 16. Living cells of the hair cortex are gradually changing into fully keratinized cortex, losing their long and thin nuclei (between *arrows*).
H and E, × 100

Fig. 17. Keratinized inner root sheath. The three layers of the inner root sheath are changing into a fused keratın substance.
H and E, × 320

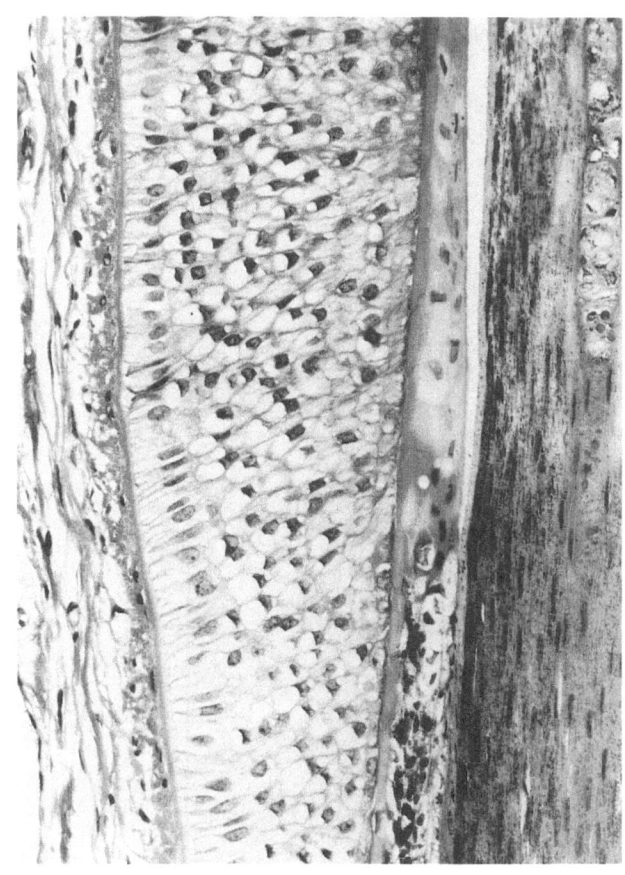

Trichilemmal keratinization

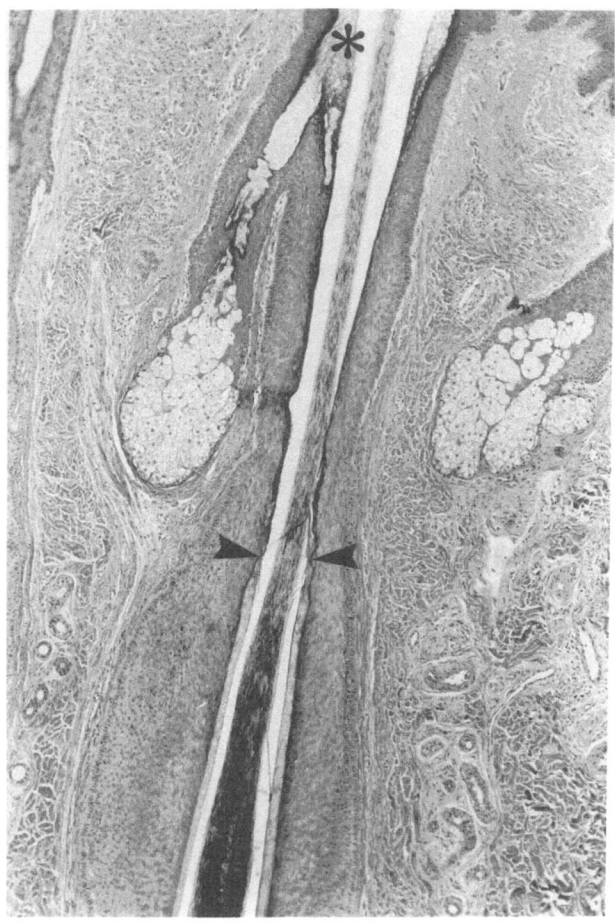

Fig. 18. This figure shows the zone of the hair follicle, extending from the free ends of the disintegrated inner root sheath (*arrows*) to the entrance of the sebaceous duct (*asterisk*). In this range, the outer root sheath shows a special type of keratinization without the formation of keratohyaline granules (trichilemmal keratinization). H and E, ×64

Fig. 19. Higher magnification. Bulky cells of the outer root sheath are protruding into the hair canal. No keratohyaline granules are seen. *Arrows* point to free ends of the inner root sheath.
H and E, × 200

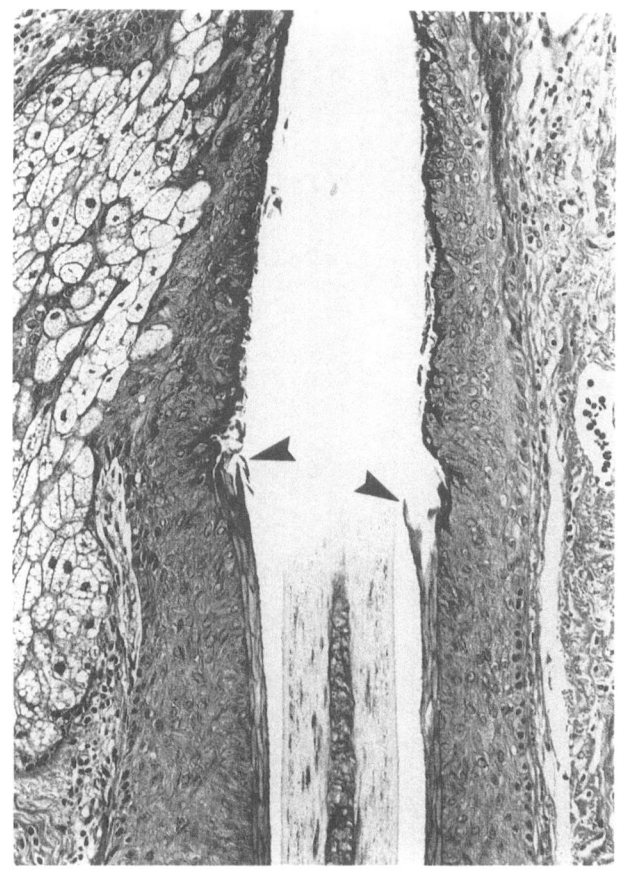

REFERENCES

1 Holmes EJ (1968) Tumors of lower hair sheath: Common histogenesis of certain so-called "sebaceous cysts", acanthomas and "sebaceous carcinomas". Cancer 21: 234–248
2 Pinkus H (1968) Static and dynamic histology and histochemistry of hair growth. In: Baccaredda-Boy A, Moretti G, Frey JR (eds) Biopathology of pattern alopecia. Karger, Basel, pp 69–81
3 Pinkus H (1969) "Sebaceous cysts" are trichilemmal cysts. Arch Dermatol 99: 544–555
4 Pinkus H, Iwasaki T, Mishima Y (1981) Outer root sheath keratinization in anagen and catagen of the mammalian hair follicle. A seventh distinct type of keratinization in the hair follicle: trichilemmal keratinization. J Anat 133: 19–35

21

Sebaceous duct

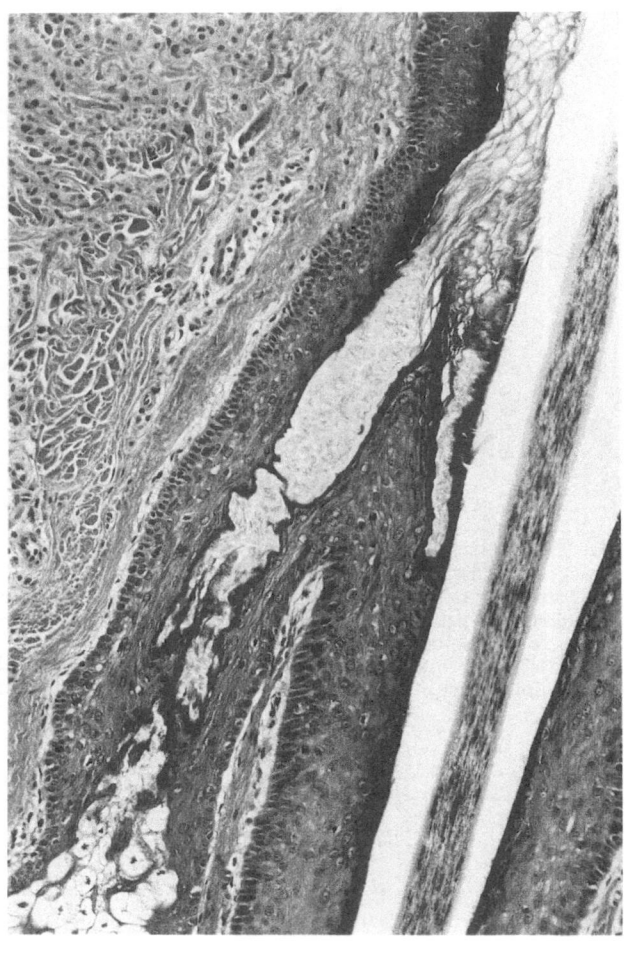

Fig. 20. Overall appearance
of a sebaceous duct.
H and E, × 160

Fig. 21. Higher magnification of Fig. 20. Keratohyaline granules are seen in the horny layer of the duct epithelium. A crenulated pattern of the horny layer as in steatocystoma is noted.
H and E, × 320

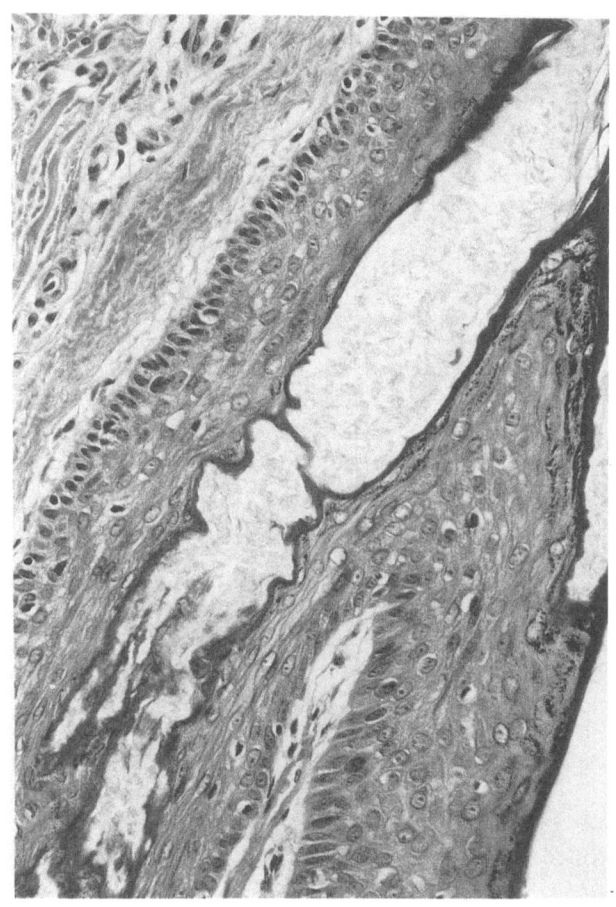

REFERENCES

1 Pinkus H, Mehregan AH (1981) A guide to dermatohistopathology, 3rd edn. Appleton-Century-Crofts, New York, pp 29, 436
2 Strauss JS, Pochi PE (1968) Histology, histochemistry, and electron microscopy of sebaceous glands in man. In: Marchionini A (ed) Handbuch der Haut- und Geschlechtskrankheiten, Ergänzungswerk, vol. 1, part 1. Springer, Berlin, pp 184–223

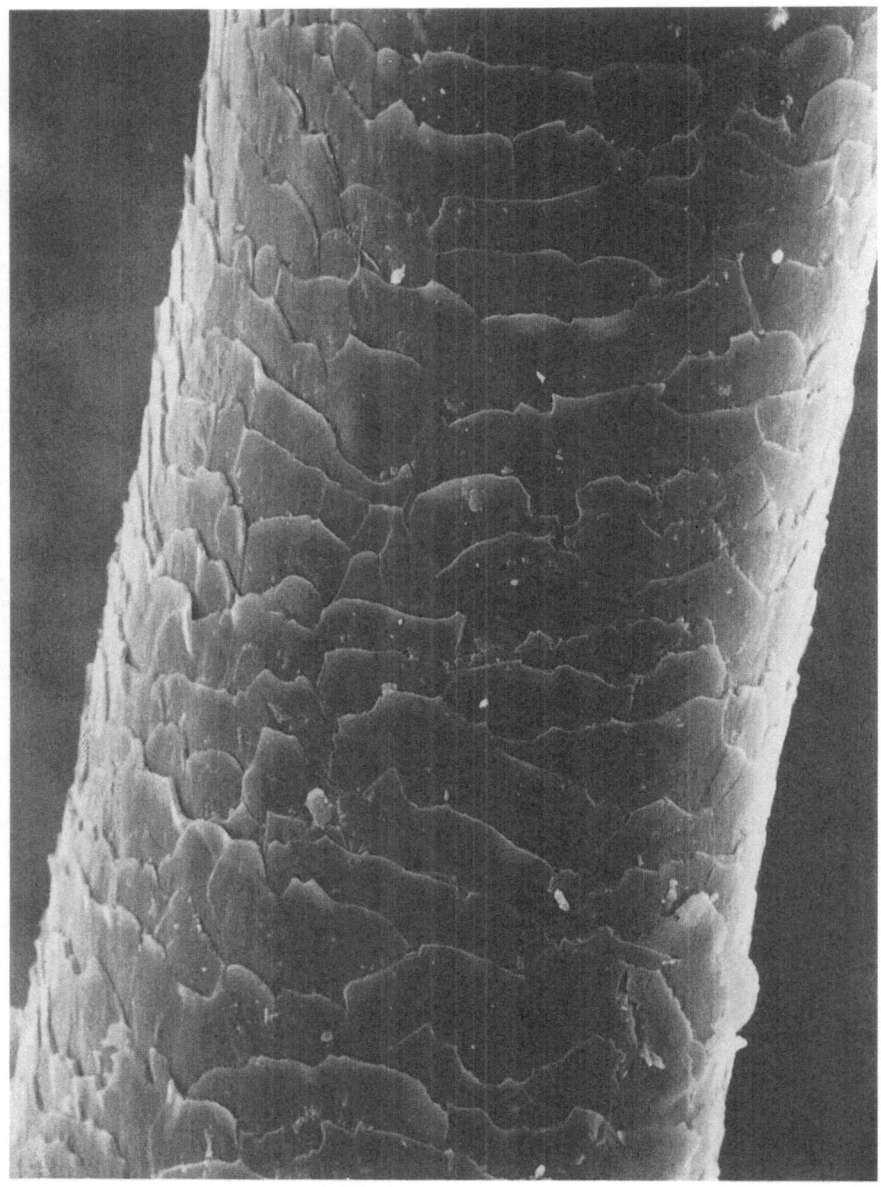

Fig. 22. Scanning electron micrograph of the hair. The outside of the hair is covered with the keratinized cuticle cells of the hair like the scales of a fish.
× 1500

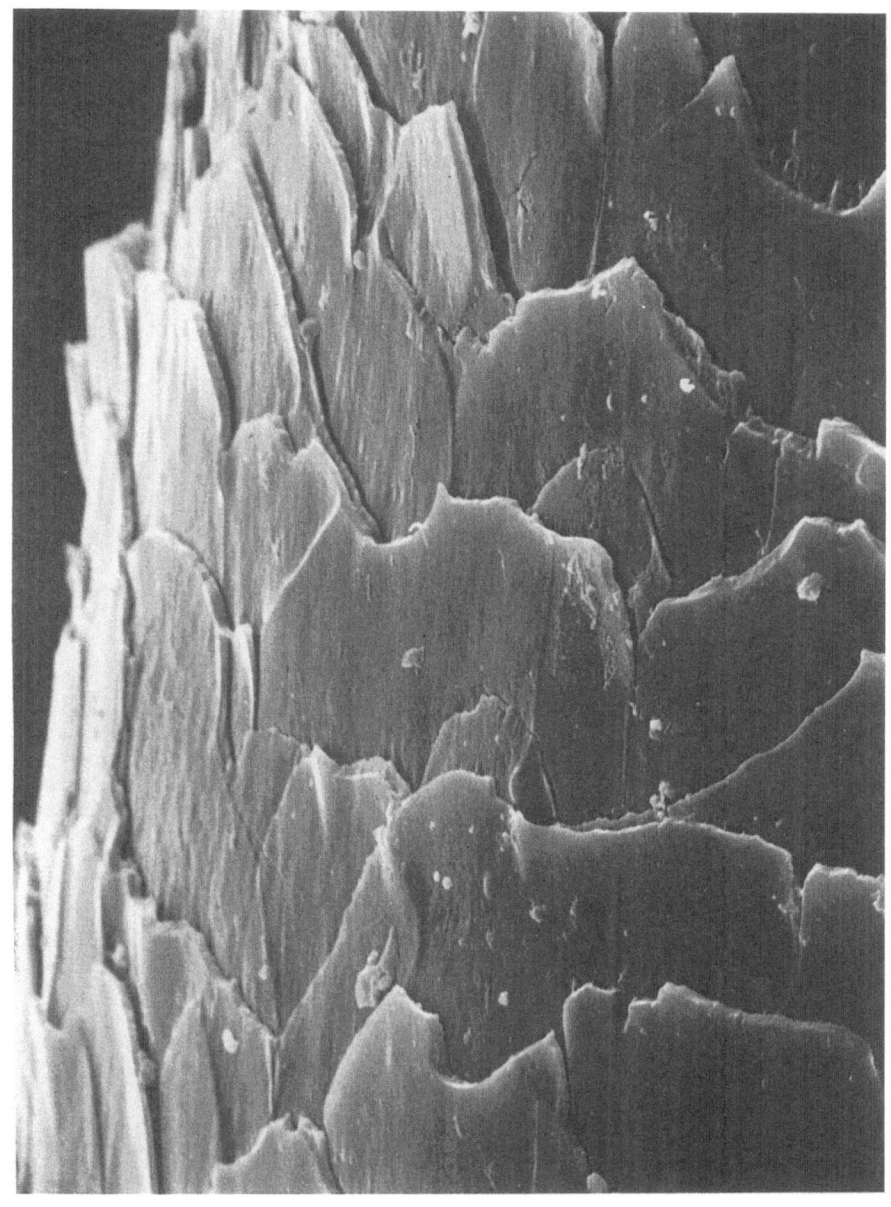

Fig. 23. Higher magnification.
×4500 (courtesy of Dr. Yasuhıro Matsumoto, Tsurumi University, School of Dentistry)

Hair cycle

Catagen follicle

The following are regarded as signs of the early catagen follicle: (1) Thickening of the glassy membrane and the fibrous root sheath, (2) loss of metachromasia of the dermal papilla, (3) cessation of melanogenesis, (4) stop of mitotic activity in the matrix, (5) shrinkage of the matrix and the dermal papilla, and (6) scattered appearance of apoptotic cells in the outer root sheath.

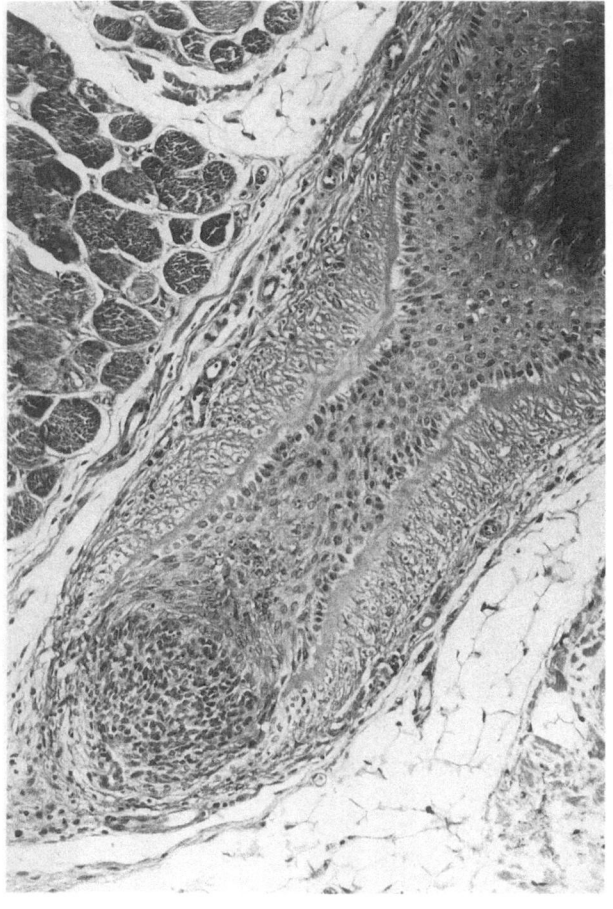

Fig. 24. The hair-cycling portion of the follicle is being retracted. Marked thickening of the fibrous root sheath is seen.
H and E, × 160

Fig. 25. Advanced catagen follicle. The fibrous root sheath is very thick and the glassy membrane is also thick and corrugated.
H and E, × 200

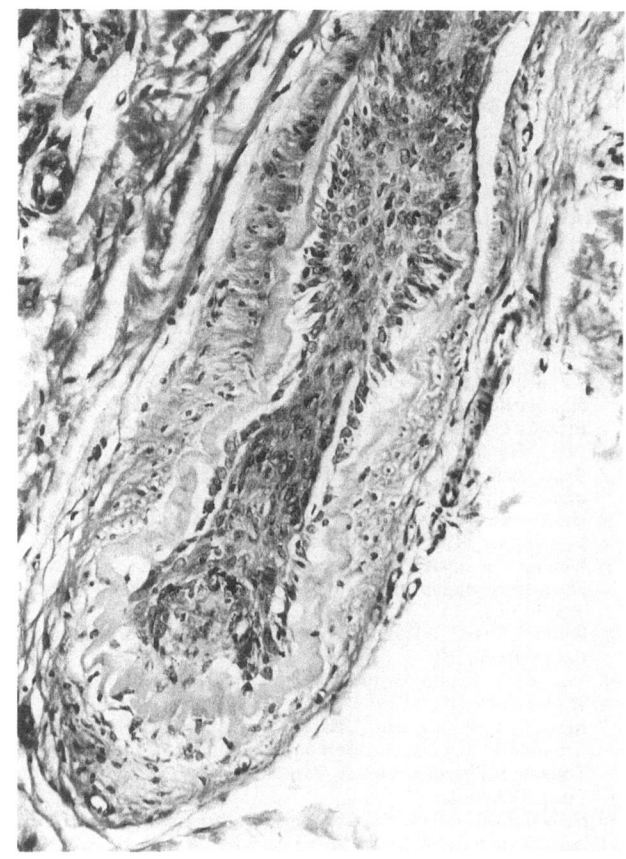

REFERENCES

1 Headington JT (1984) Transverse microscopic anatomy of the human scalp: A basis for a morphometric approach to disorders of the hair follicle. Arch Dermatol 120: 449–456
2 Kligman AM (1959) The human hair cycle. J Invest Dermatol 33: 307–316
3 Montagna W (1962) The structure and function of skin, 2nd edn. Academic Press, New York, pp 196–209
4 Olson RL, Everett MA (1975) Epidermal apoptosis: Cell deletion by phagocytosis. J Cutan Pathol 2: 53–57
5 Pinkus H (1980) Factors in the formation of club hair. In: Brown AC, Crounse RG (eds) Hair, trace elements, and human illness. Praeger, New York, pp 147–154
6 Weedon D, Strutton G (1981) Apoptosis as the mechanism of the involution of hair follicles in catagen transformation. Acta Derm Venereol (Stockh) 61: 335–339
7 Weedon D, Strutton G (1984) The recognition of early stages of catagen. Am J Dermatopathol 6: 553–555

Trichilemmal sac (Pinkus), Haarbeet (Unna), Kolbenlager (Auburtin)

The catagen hair follicle is retracted to the base of the trichilemmal sac, which is the lower portion of the permanent hair follicle, and in which the club hair is anchored. The cells of the trichilemmal sac show the same keratinization as that of the isthmus zone of the anagen hair follicle (Figs. 18, 19). It is occasionally seen in the epidermal keratinization of tumors, such as cutaneous horn [2, 7, 10, 12], trichilemmal keratosis [5], trichilemmoma [3], seborrheic keratosis [8, 11], keratoacanthoma [9], wart [6], and verrucous trichilemmal tumor [9] and in onycholemmal horn [4].

REFERENCES

1 Auburtin G (1896) Das Vorkommen von Kolbenhaaren und die Veränderungen derselben beim Haarwiederersatz, Arch Mikrosk Anat 47: 472–500
2 Brownstein MH (1979) Trichilemmal horn: cutaneous horn showing trichilemmal keratinization. Br J Dermatol 100: 303–309
3 Brownstein MH, Shapiro EE (1979) Trichilemmomal horn: cutaneous horn overlying trichilemmoma. Clin Exp Dermatol 4: 59–63
4 Haneke E (1983) 'Onycholemmal' horn. Dermatologica 167: 155–158
5 Headington JT (1976) Tumors of the hair follicle: A review. Am J Pathol 85: 480–514
6 Kimura S, Komatsu T, Ohyama K (1982) Common and plantar warts with trichilemmal keratinization-like keratinizing process: a possible existence of pseudo-trichilemmal keratinization. J Cutan Pathol 9: 391–395
7 Kimura S (1983) Trichilemmal keratosis (horn): a light and electron microscopic study. J Cutan Pathol 10: 59–67
8 Masuda M, Kimura S (1984) Trichilemmal keratinization in seborrheic keratoses. J Cutan Pathol 11: 12–17
9 Morioka S, Yamaguchi Z, Baba S, Koura T (1976) Follicular tumors and cysts: On the characteristics and the diagnostic value of keratohyaline granules seen in hair follicles and outer root sheath. In: Toda K, Ishibashi Y, Hori Y, Morikawa F (eds) Biology and disease of the hair. University of Tokyo Press, Tokyo, pp 377–396
10 Nakamura K (1984) Two cases of trichilemmal-like horn. Arch Dermatol 120: 386–387
11 Nakayasu K, Nishimura A, Maruo M, Wakabayashi S (1981) Trichilemmal differentiation in seborrheic keratosis. J Cutan Pathol 8: 256–262
12 Peteiro MC, Toribio J. Caeiro JL (1984) Trichilemmal horn. J Cutan Pathol 11: 326–328
13 Pinkus F (1927) Die normale Anatomie der Haut. In: Jadassohn J (ed) Handbuch der Haut- und Geschlechtskrankheiten, vol. 1, part 1. Springer, Berlin, pp 212–217
14 Pinkus H, Mehregan AH (1981) A guide to dermatohistopathology, 3rd edn. Appleton-Century-Crofts, New York, pp 25–32
15 Unna P (1876) Beiträge zur Histologie und Entwickelungsgeschichte der menschlichen Oberhaut und ihrer Anhangsgebilde. Arch Mikrosk Anat 12: 665–741

Fig. 26. Keratinizing cells of the outer root sheath are converging into the catagen club hair, without the formation of keratohyaline granules. H and E, × 200

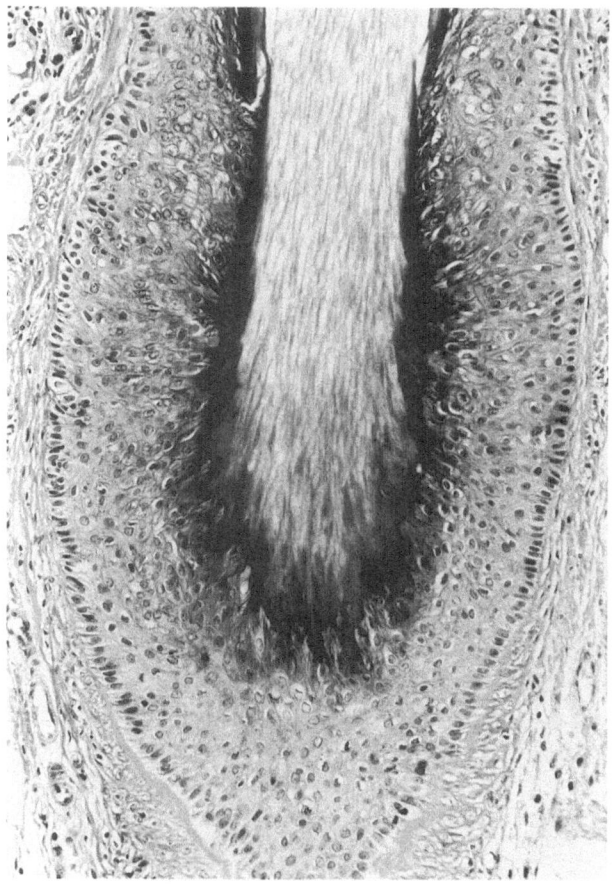

Early anagen follicle

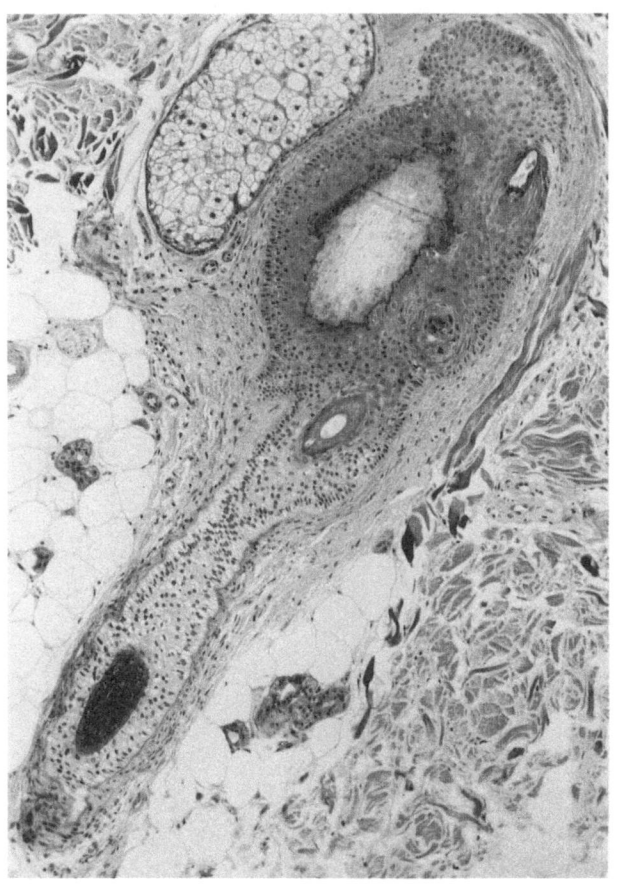

Fig. 27. An early anagen follicle found in a section of seborrheic keratosis in the preauricular region of a 69-year-old woman. From the right side of the base of the trichilemmal sac, the new anagen follicle is growing downward and upward alongside the old club hair.
H and E, × 100

Fig. 28. Higher magnification ▷ of Fig. 27. The hair and the inner root sheath are seen in the glycogen-rich new hair follicle.
H and E, × 200

Fig. 29. Higher magnification ▷ of Fig. 27. The tip of the hair is seen in the new hair canal (*arrow*).
H and E, × 200

REFERENCES

1 Auburtin G (1896) Das Vorkommen von Kolbenhaaren und die Veränderungen derselben beim Haarwiederersatz. Arch Mikrosk Anat 47: 472–500
2 Ioannides G (1982) Alopecia: A pathologist's view. Int J Dermatol 21: 316–328
3 Kligman AM (1961) Pathologic dynamics of human hair loss: I. Telogen effluvium. Arch Dermatol 83: 175–198
4 Pinkus F (1927) Die normale Anatomie der Haut. In: Jadassohn J (ed) Handbuch der Haut- und Geschlechtskrankheiten, vol. 1, part 1. Springer, Berlin, pp 212–217
5 Pinkus H, Mehregan AH (1981) A guide to dermatohistopathology, 3rd edn. Appleton-Century-Crofts, New York, pp 31–32
6 Price ML, Griffiths WAD (1985) Normal body hair—a review. Clin Exp Dermatol 10: 87–97
7 Rook A, Dawber R (1982) Diseases of the hair and scalp. Blackwell, Oxford, pp 9–17
8 Sato Y (1976) The hair cycle and its control mechanism. In: Toda K, Ishibashi Y, Hori Y, Morikawa F (eds) Biology and disease of the hair. University of Tokyo Press, Tokyo, pp 3–13
9 Unna P (1876) Beiträge zur Histologie und Entwickelungsgeschichte der menschlichen Oberhaut und ihrer Anhangsgebilde. Arch Mikrosk Anat 12: 665–741
10 Uno H, Cappas A, Schlagel C (1985) Cyclic dynamics of hair follicles and the effect of minoxidil on the bald scalps of stumptailed macaques. Am J Dermatopathol 7: 283–297

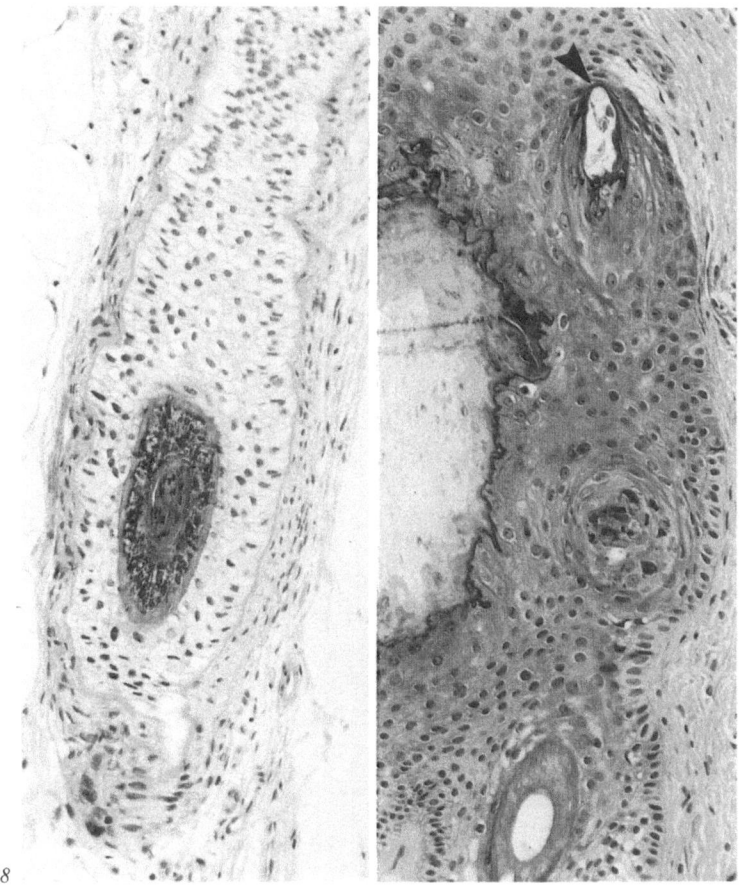

28   29

31

Arao-Perkins body

An elastinlike body is noted at the entrance to the dermal papilla. It remains at this site during the catagen stage; the next anagen follicle grows down to this body. To demonstrate this material, acid orcein or resorcinol fuchsin must be used [5–7].

REFERENCES

1 Arao T, Perkins EM Jr (1969) The interrelation of elastic tissue and human hair follicles. In: Montagna W, Dobson RL (eds) Advances in biology of skin, vol IX. Hair growth. Pergamon, Oxford, pp 433–440
2 Arao T, Perkins EM Jr (1970) The relation between hair growth cycle and the development of elastic fibers in the connective tissue sheath of hair follicles. Jpn J Dermatol Ser B 80: 245–248
3 Arao T (1976) Connective tissue hair sheath especially on the structure and development of elastic tissues. In: Toda K, Ishibashi Y, Hori Y, Morikawa F (eds) Biology and disease of the hair. University of Tokyo Press, Tokyo, pp 15–22
4 Pinkus H (1978) Epithelial-mesodermal interaction in normal hair growth, alopecia, and neoplasia. J Dermatol (Tokyo) 5: 93–101
5 Pinkus H (1978) Differential patterns of elastic fibers in scarring and non-scarring alopecias. J Cutan Pathol 5: 93–104
6 Pinkus H (1980) Alopecia: Clinicopathologic correlations. Int J Dermatol 19: 245–253
7 Pinkus H (1981) Alterations of the hair follicle in hair diseases. In: Orfanos CE, Montagna W, Stüttgen G (eds) Hair research: Status and future aspects. Springer, Berlin, pp 237–243
8 Pinkus H, Mehregan AH (1981) A guide to dermatohistopathology, 3rd edn. Appleton-Century-Crofts, New York, pp 28, 214–215, 547–548

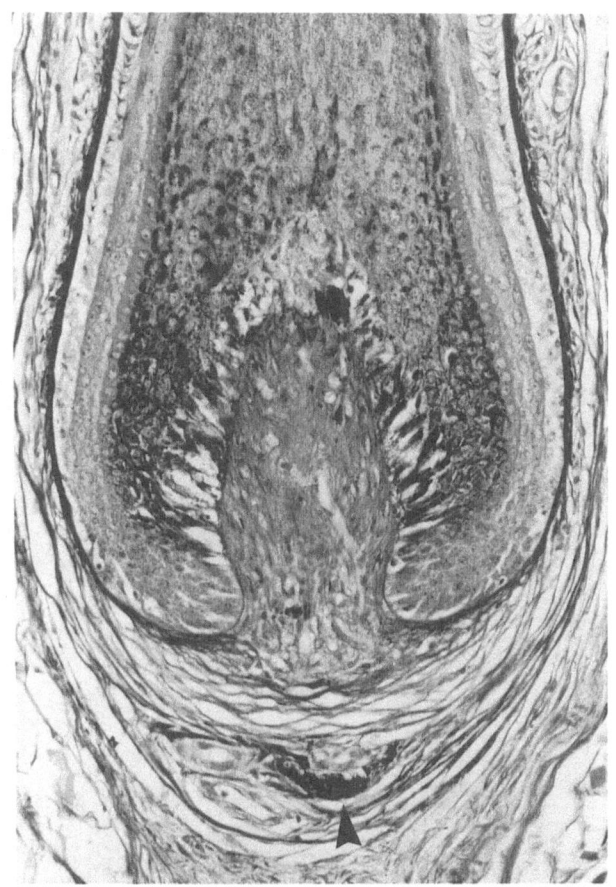

Arrector pili muscle

The arrector pili muscle is attached to the bulge (*Wulst*), a swelling on the posterior side of the hair follicle, to the level of which the hair-cycling portion of a follicle disintegrates in the catagen stage. The zone of the hair canal from this site to the entrance of the sebaceous duct is called the isthmus.

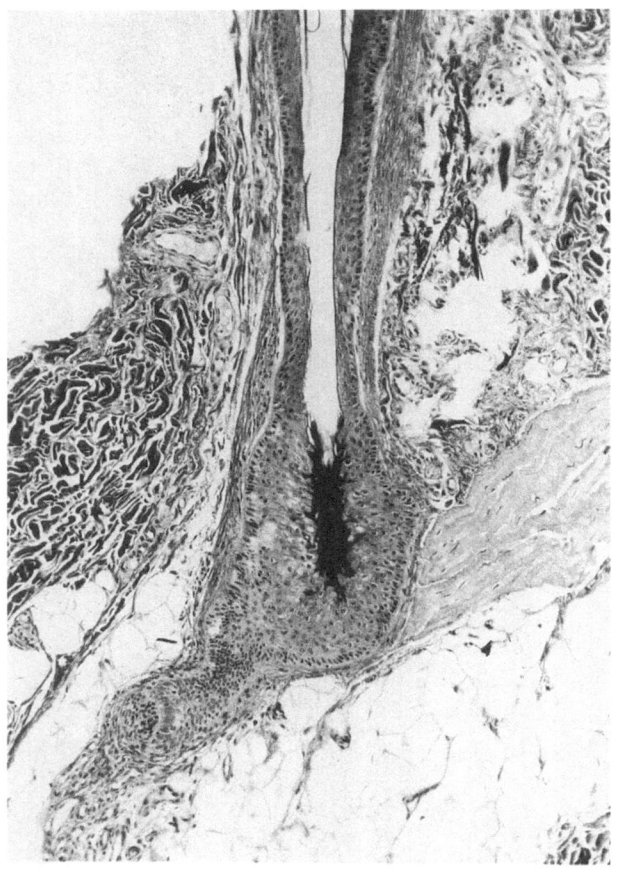

Fig. 31. The arrector pili muscle is seen fixed to the bulge. A presumptive early anagen follicle is growing from the base of the trichilemmal sac.
H and E, × 100

Fig. 32. High magnification
of Fig. 31. Mitosis is seen in
the matrix of the early anagen follicle (*arrow*).
H and E, × 400

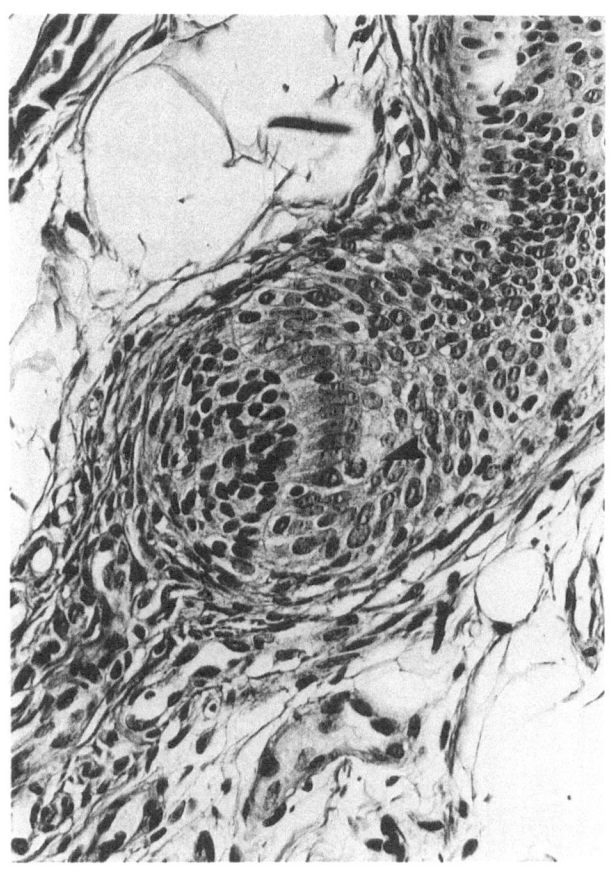

REFERENCES

1 Kanaizuka Z (1926) Beiträge zur Morphologie des Musculus arrector pili. Folia Anat Jpn 4: 141–169
2 Pinkus F (1927) Die normale Anatomie der Haut. In: Jadassohn J (ed) Handbuch der Haut- und
  Geschlechtskrankheiten, vol. 1, part 1. Springer, Berlin, pp 116–122, 256–266
3 Pinkus H, Mehregan AH (1981) A guide to dermatohistopathology, 3rd edn. Appleton-Century-
  Crofts, New York, pp 22–32

Sebaceous follicle of face

REFERENCES

1 Kligman AM, Shelley WB (1958) An investigation of the biology of the human sebaceous gland. J Invest Dermatol 30: 99–125
2 Pinkus H, Mehregan AH (1981) A guide to dermatohistopathology, 3rd edn. Appleton-Century-Crofts, New York, pp 24–25
3 Strauss JS, Pochi PE (1968) Histology, histochemistry, and electron microscopy of sebaceous glands in man. In: Marchionini A (ed) Handbuch der Hant- und Geschlechtskrankheiten, Ergänzungswerk, vol. 1, part 1. Springer, Berlin, pp 184–223

Fig. 33. Because of hyper-
trophied sebaceous glands,
the lower portion of hair follicle is pushed aside as if it
were an appendage to the
pilary complex.
H and E, × 100

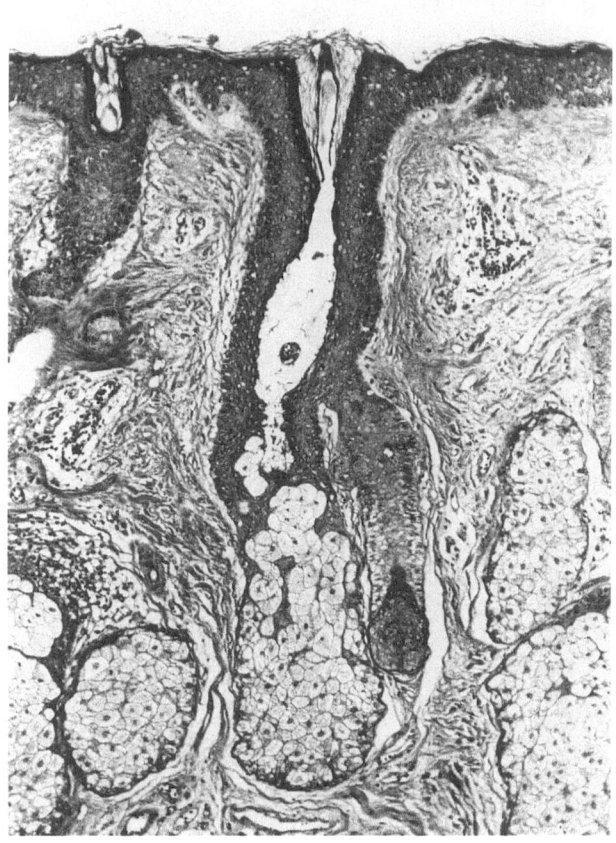

Compound follicles

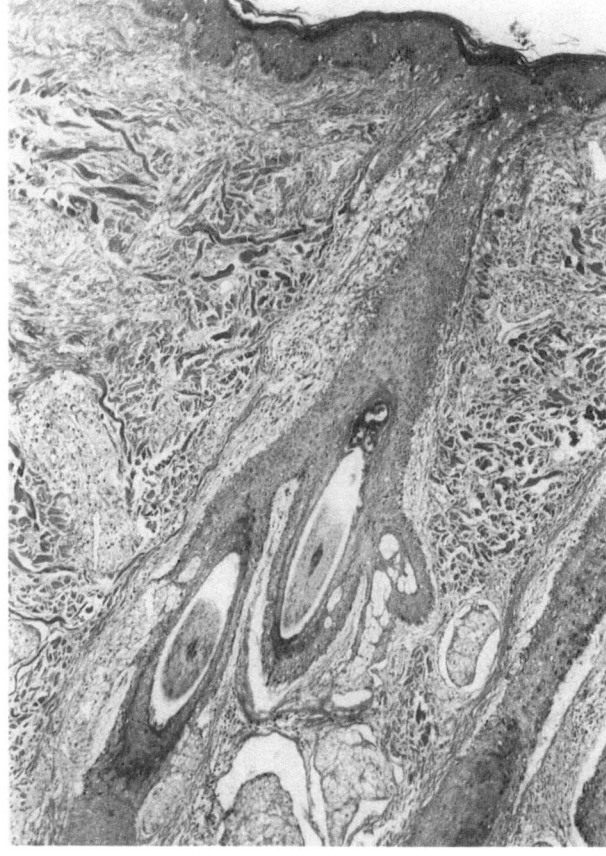

Fig. 34. Two hair follicles are joining.
H and E, × 64

Fig. 35. Two anagen follicles of vellus hair type are entering a common hair canal. H and E, × 160

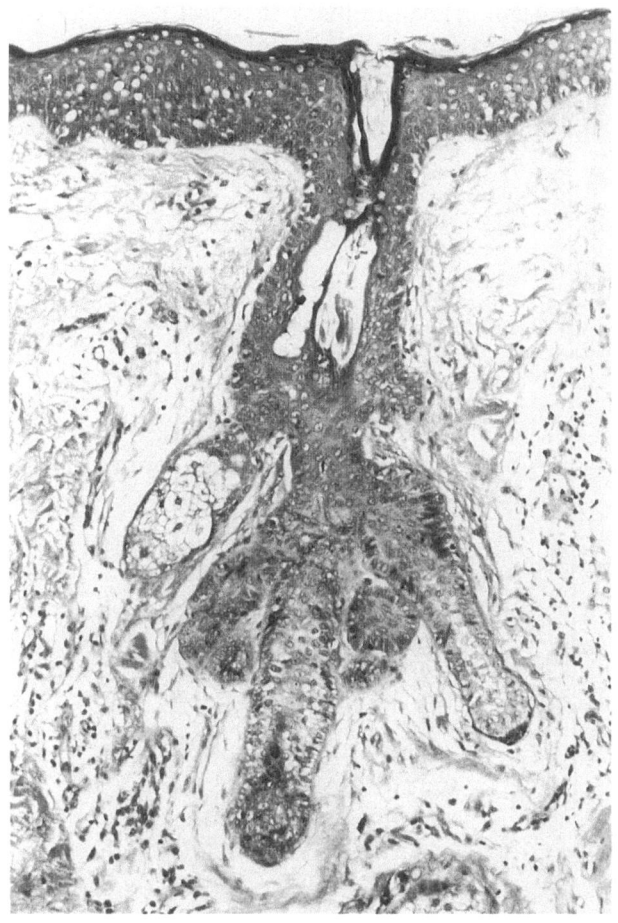

REFERENCES

1 Loewenthal LJA (1947) "Compound" and grouped hairs of the human scalp: Their possible connection with follicular infections. J Invest Dermatol 8: 263–273
2 Oberste-Lehn H (1957) Die Bedeutung der Bündelhaare im menschlichen Haarkleid für die chronischen Follikulitiden. Arch Klin Exp Dermatol 206: 506–512
3 Oberste-Lehn H, Nobis A (1963) Die Haaranordnung beim Menschen und bei einigen Säugetieren. Z Anat Entwicklungsgesch 123: 589–642
4 Pinkus H (1951) Multiple hairs (Flemming-Giovannini): Report of two cases of pili multigemini and discussion of some other anomalies of the pilary complex. J Invest Dermatol 17: 291–301

Mantle hair, Mantelhaar (F. Pinkus)

This type of vellus hair follicle is not infrequently found in routine sections. The mantle hair is a bell-shaped structure of rudimentary sebaceous glands surrounding the follicle.

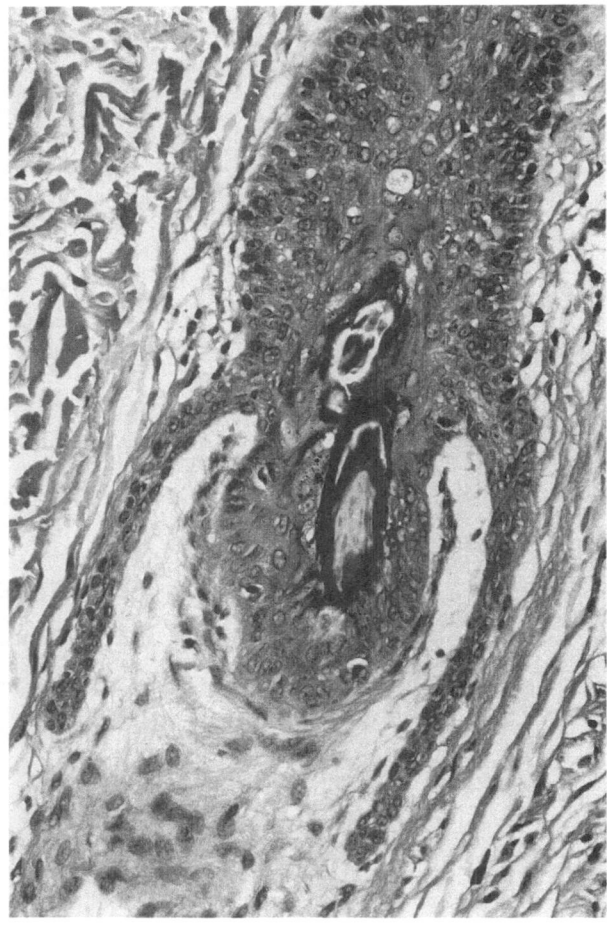

Fig. 36. In longitudinal section, thin epithelial cords are seen on both sides of the hair follicle.
H and E, × 320

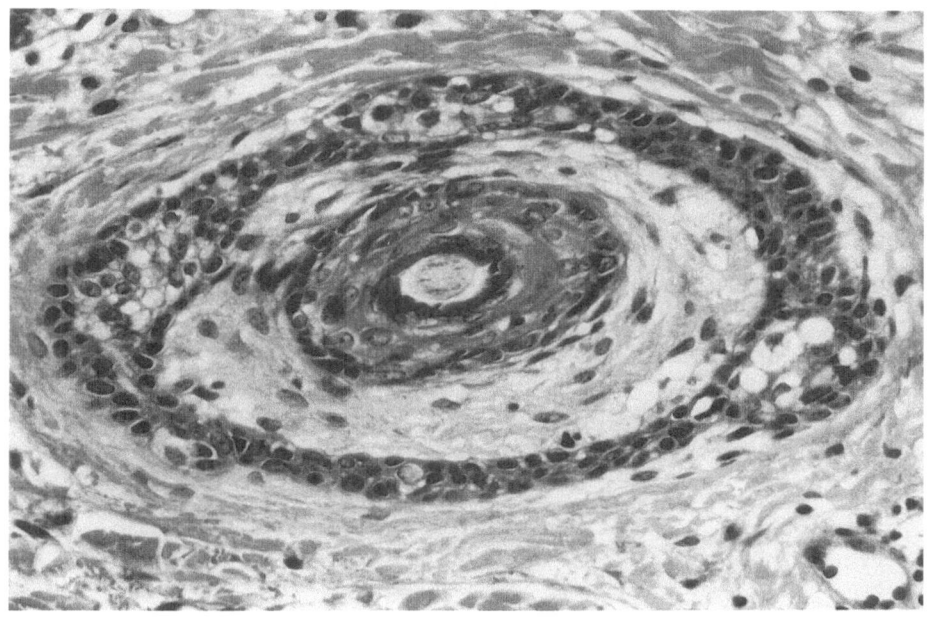

Fig. 37. In cross section, the cords appear as a closed epithelial ring encircling the hair follicle. Sebaceous cells are seen in the ring.
H and E, × 400

REFERENCES

1 Epstein W, Kligman AM (1956) The pathogenesis of milia and benign tumors of the skin. J Invest Dermatol 26: 1–11
2 Pinkus F (1897) Ueber eine Form rudimentärer Talgdrüsen. Arch Dermatol Syph (Berl) 41: 347–356
3 Pinkus H, Mehregan AH (1981) A guide to dermatohistopathology, 3rd edn. Appleton-Century-Crofts, New York, pp 29, 211, 274

Basal cell epitheliomalike changes of hair follicle in dermatofibroma

REFERENCES

1 Goette DK, Helwig EB (1975) Basal cell carcinomas and basal cell carcinoma-like changes overlying dermatofibromas. Arch Dermatol 111: 589–592
2 Korom I, Simon N (1984) Epithelveränderungen beim Dermatofibrom. Z Hautkr 59: 969–974
3 Pinkus H (1967) Pathobiology of the pilary complex. Jpn J Dermatol Ser B 77: 304–330
4 Pinkus H, Mehregan AH (1981) A guide to dermatohistopathology, 3rd edn. Appleton-Century-Crofts, New York, pp 273–275
5 Rahbari H, Mehregan AH (1985) Adnexal displacement and regression in association with histiocytoma (dermatofibroma). J Cutan Pathol 12: 94–102
6 Steigleder GK, Nicklas H, Kamei Y (1962) Die Epithelveränderungen beim Histiozytom, ihre Genese und ihr Erscheinungsbild. Dermatol Wochenschr 146: 457–468

Fig. 39. Higher magnification of Fig. 38. ▷
H and E, × 160

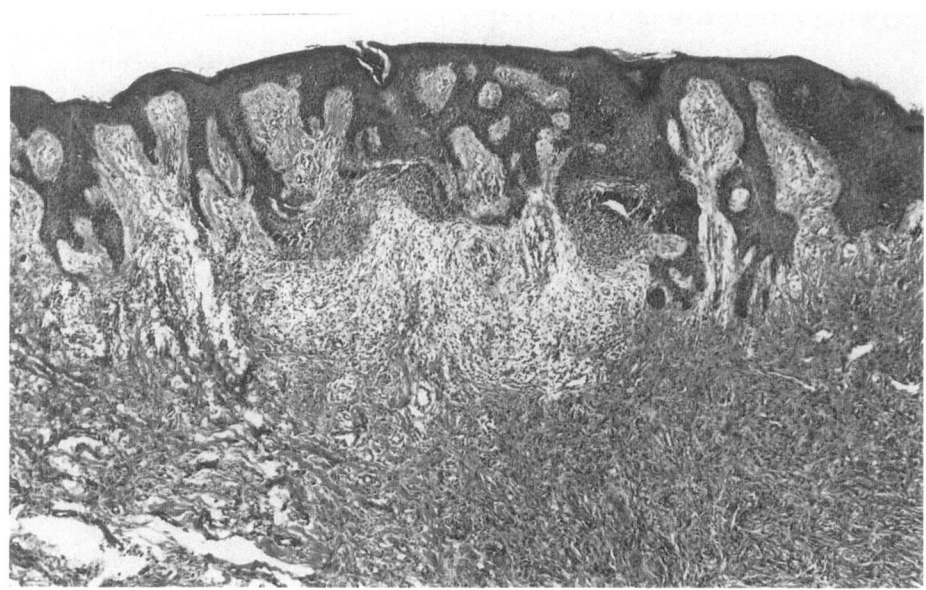

Fig. 38. At first glance, a superficial basal cell epithelioma seems to be arising from the epidermis. But on close examination, the mesenchymal cells, like those of the dermal papilla, are seen massed around the basaloid cells in three places. These changes are interpreted as being caused by regression of the hair follicles, downward growth of which has been suppressed by proliferation of dermatofibroma. H and E, ×64

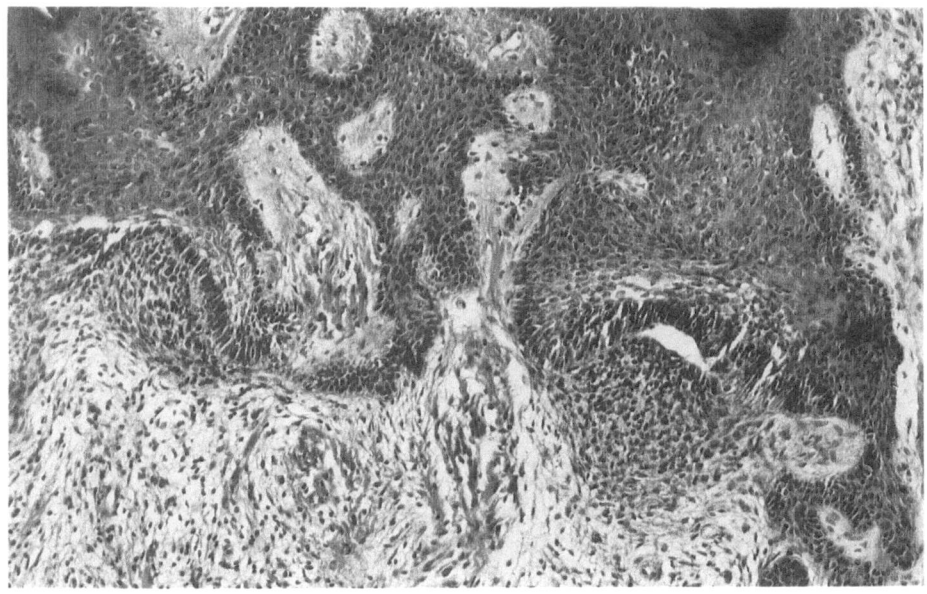

APOCRINE GLANDS

The secretory portion of the apocrine glands shows a complicated coiling, making shunts between adjacent coils and, in other places, diverticula. In contrast to eccrine glands, the secretory portion consists of only one type of cell surrounded by an outer layer of myoepithelial cells. The secretory cells show decapitation secretion. According to an electron-microscopic study of Schaumburg-Lever and Lever, there are three types of secretion in the apocrine glands—merocrine, apocrine, and holocrine [9]. Acid-fast bodies, which are seen in the eccrine glands, are also found in the apocrine glands [8].

REFERENCES

1 Braun-Falco O, Rupec M (1968) Apokrine Schweißdrüsen. In: Marchionini A (ed) Handbuch der Haut- und Geschlechtskrankheiten, Ergänzungswerk, vol. 1, part 1. Springer, Berlin, pp 267–338

2 Craigmyle MBL (1984) The apocrine glands and the breast. Wiley, Chichester, pp 9–31

3 Hurley HJ, Shelley WB (1960) The human apocrine sweat gland in health and disease. Thomas, Springfield, IL, pp 2, 6–21

4 Inoue T (1979) Scanning electron microscopic study of the human axillary apocrine glands. J Dermatol (Tokyo) 6: 299–308

5 Kurosumi K, Kurosumi U (1982) Further studies on the ultrastructure of the human axillary apocrine sweat glands. Okajimas Folia Anat Jpn 58: 305–323

6 Montagna W (1962) The structure and function of skin, 2nd edn. Academic Press, New York, pp 374–424

7 Pinkus H (1964) Die makroskopische Anatomie der Haut. In: Marchionini A (ed) Handbuch der Haut- und Geschlechtskrankheiten, Ergänzungswerk, vol. 1, part 2. Springer, Berlin, pp 21–24

8 Rahbari H (1980) Acid fast bodies in eccrine and apocrine sweat glands. J Cutan Pathol 7: 342–348

9 Schaumburg-Lever G, Lever WF (1975) Secretion from human apocrine glands: An electron microscopic study. J Invest Dermatol 64: 38–41

10 Schiefferdecker P (1917) Die Hautdrüsen des Menschen und der Säugetiere, ihre biologische und rassenanatomische Bedeutung sowie die Muscularis sexualis. Biol Zentralbl 37: 534–562

11 Smith JD, Hearn GW (1979) Ultrastructure of the apocrine-sebaceous anal scent gland of the woodchuck, *Marmota monax*: Evidence for apocrine and merocrine secretion by a single cell type. Anat Rec 193: 269–291

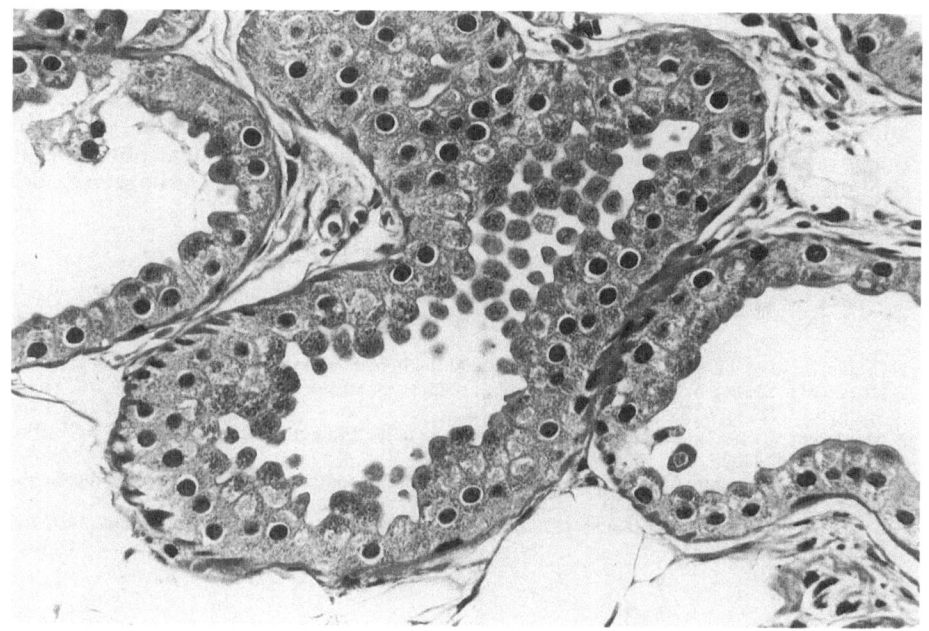

Fig. 40. Marked decapitation secretion is noted in the secretory cells.
H and E, × 400

Apocrine duct

Since the apocrine glands originate from the primary epithelial germ (Marks), the apocrine duct belongs to the hair follicle (apo-pilo sebaceous unit). The intradermal apocrine duct is straight and follows a course close to the hair follicle. It opens into the infundibulum and, unlike the acrosyringium, the intrafollicular portion is also straight. It is not infrequent for two or occasionally three ducts to be seen entering the same follicle [2].

REFERENCES

1 Craigmyle MBL (1984) The apocrine glands and the breast. Wiley, Chichester, pp 9–16, 20
2 Hurley HJ, Shelley WB (1960) The human apocrine sweat gland in health and disease. Thomas, Springfield, IL, pp 6–23
3 Montagna W (1962) The structure and function of skin, 2nd edn. Academic Press, New York, pp 374–377, 400–402
4 Pinkus H, Mehregan AH (1981) A guide to dermatohistopathology, 3rd edn. Appleton-Century-Crofts, New York, pp 6, 29–30
5 Tani M, Yamamoto K, Mishima Y (1980) Apocrine acrosyringeal complex in the human skin. J Invest Dermatol 75: 431–435

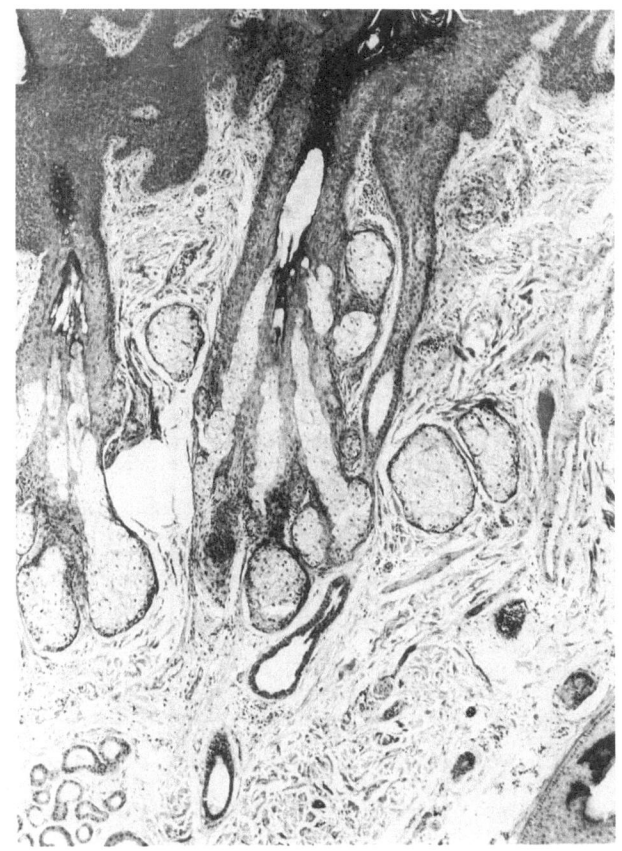

Fig. 41. A straight apocrine duct is seen running close to the hair follicle and opening into the ınfundibulum.
H and E, ×64

ECCRINE GLANDS

Since the eccrine glands are merocrine in nature, they discharge sweat without loss of the cytoplasm. Ito was the first to recognize two kinds of cell in the secretory portion—"superficial" and "basal" cells [2, 3]. The former are now generally termed dark cells, and the latter clear cells. The clear cells are larger and secrete aqueous material; the dark cells are smaller and secrete mucin. Between the clear cells, there are intercellular canaliculi, through which sweat from the clear cells empties into the lumina. In addition, myoepithelial cells, which are capable of contraction, are found at the base of the secretory portion. Acid-fast granules are found in the secretory cells [10].

REFERENCES

1 Ellis RA (1968) Eccrine sweat glands: Electron microscopy, cytochemistry and anatomy. In: Marchionini A (ed) Handbuch der Haut- und Geschlechtskrankheiten, Ergänzungswerk, vol. 1, part 1. Springer, Berlin, pp 224–266
2 Ito T (1943) Über den Golgiapparat der ekkrinen Schweißdrüsenzellen der menschlichen Haut. Okajimas Folia Anat Jpn 22: 273–280
3 Ito T, Iwashige K (1951) Zytologische Untersuchung über die ekkrinen Schweißdrüsen in menschlicher Achselhaut mit besonderer Berücksichtigung der apokrinen Sekretion derselben. Okajimas Folia Anat Jpn 23: 147–166
4 Ito T, Shibasaki S (1966) Electron microscopic study on human eccrine sweat glands. Arch Histol Jpn 27: 81–115
5 Kurosumi K, Kurosumi U, Tosaka H (1982) Ultrastructure of human eccrine sweat glands with special reference to the transitional portion. Arch Histol Jpn 45: 213–238
6 Lee MMC (1960) Histology and histochemistry of human eccrine sweat glands, with special reference to their defense mechanisms. Anat Rec 136: 97–105
7 Lever WF, Schaumburg-Lever G (1983) Histopathology of the skin, 6th edn. Lippincott, Philadelphia, pp 20–22
8 Montagna W, Chase HB, Lobitz WC Jr (1953) Histology and cytochemistry of human skin: IV. The eccrine sweat glands. J Invest Dermatol 20: 415–423
9 Montagna W (1962) The structure and function of skin, 2nd edn. Academic Press, New York, pp 312–373
10 Pinkus H, Mehregan AH (1981) A guide to dermatohistopathology, 3rd edn. Appleton-Century-Crofts, New York, pp 32–34

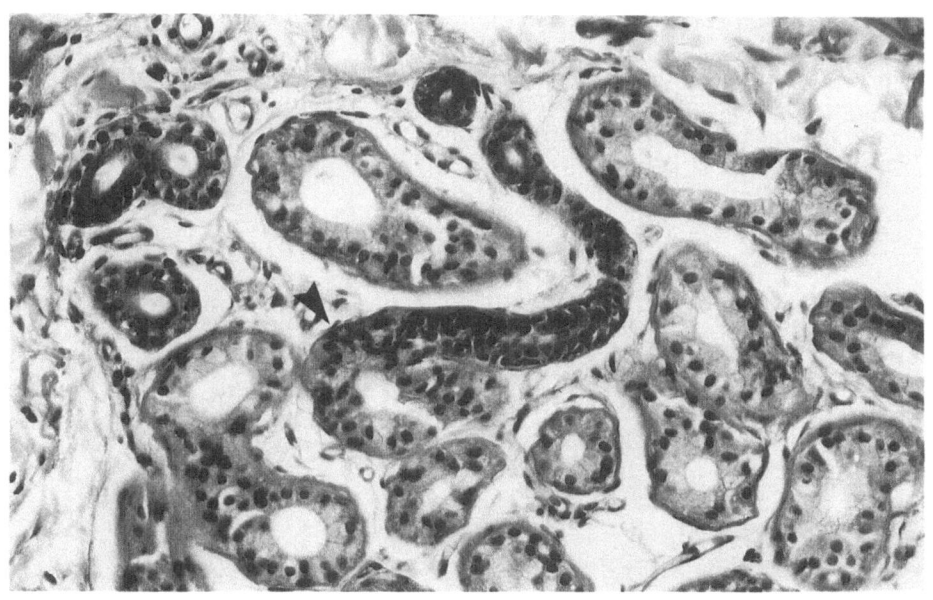

Fig. 42. A large number of secretory portions are shown. A secretory portion is seen abruptly changing into the duct (*arrow*).
H and E, × 320

Intraepidermal eccrine sweat duct unit (acrosyringium)

Since the duct ascends spirally, it is cut several times. The acrosyringium is a biologically independent unit different from the epidermis; the matrix zone of it is in the subepidermal portion of the eccrine duct [1, 4].

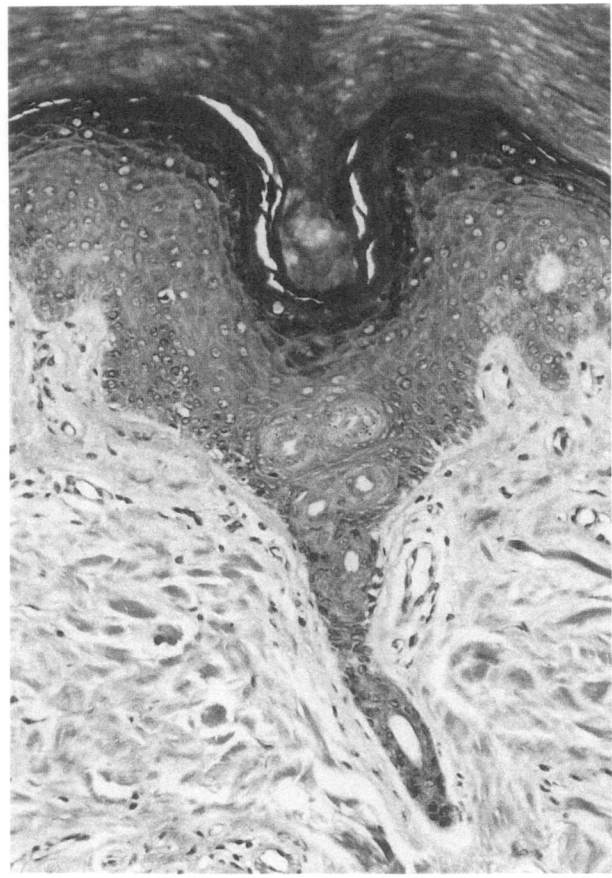

Fig. 43. Low magnification of the acrosyringium. H and E, × 200

Fig. 44. Since the cuticle-lined duct undergoes epidermoid keratinization earlier than the epidermis, keratohyaline granules appear in the middle of the epidermis.
H and E, × 400

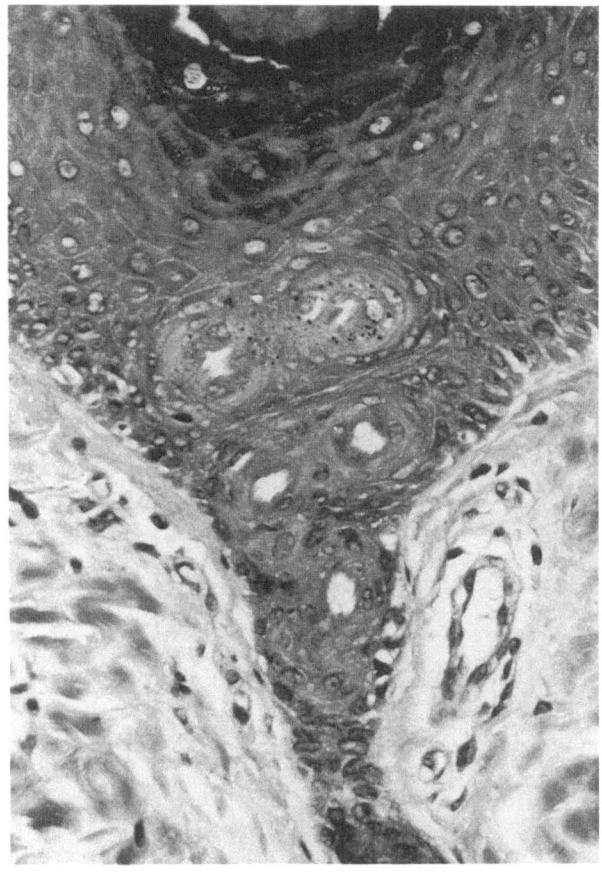

REFERENCES

1 Christophers E, Plewig G (1973) Formation of the acrosyringium. Arch Dermatol 107: 378–382
2 Lobitz WC Jr, Holyoke JB, Montagna W (1954) "The epidermal eccrine sweat duct unit": A morphologic and biologic entity. J Invest Dermatol 22: 157–158
3 Pinkus H (1939) Notes on the anatomy and pathology of the skin appendages: I. The wall of the intra-epidermal part of the sweat duct. J Invest Dermatol 2: 175–186
4 Pinkus H, Mehregan AH (1981) A guide to dermatohistopathology, 3rd edn. Appleton-Century-Crofts, New York, pp 15–16, 32–34

Intradermal eccrine sweat duct

REFERENCE

Wells TR, Landing BH (1968) The helical course of the human eccrine sweat duct. J Invest Dermatol 51: 177–185

Fig. 45. In this section, the intradermal sweat duct is stretched. The duct follows a basically helical course, but in a three-dimensional visualization it meanders through the dermis.
H and E, × 100

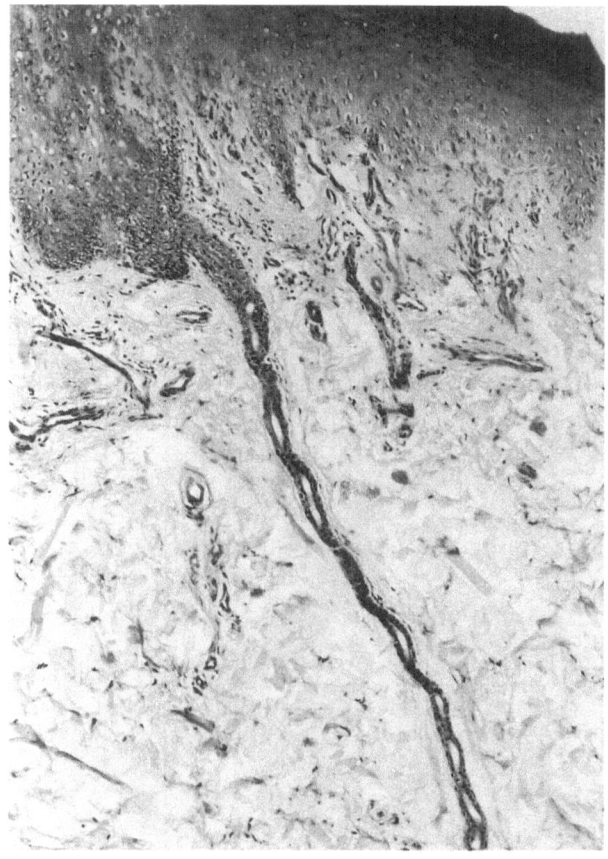

Eccrine sweat glands with clear reticulated cytoplasm

Eccrine sweat glands with clear reticulated cytoplasm were first described by Holyoke and Lobitz [5]; these glands are occasionally found in routine histological sections. Rupec noted this cytoplasmic change. From electron-microscopic studies using acid phosphatase, he concluded that there might be a mode of holocrine secretion in the cytoplasm of secretory cells of this type [9].

REFERENCES

1 Belcher RW (1973) Ultrastructure and function of eccrine glands in the mucopolysaccharidoses. Arch Pathol 96: 339–341
2 Burket JM, Brooks R, Burket DA (1985) Eccrine gland clear reticulated cytoplasm. J Am Acad Dermatol 13: 497–500
3 Drut R (1978) Eccrine sweat gland involvement in GM$_1$ gangliosidosis. J Cutan Pathol 5: 35–36
4 Grosshans E, Juillard J, Libert JP, Candas V, Vogt JJ (1980) Physiopathology of sweating response in individuals with eccrine glands of the rare reticulated clear cell type. J Invest Dermatol 74: 455–456
5 Holyoke JB, Lobitz WC Jr (1952) Histologic variations in the structure of human eccrine sweat glands. J Invest Dermatol 18: 147–167
6 Martin JJ, Ceuterick C, Martin L, Libert J (1977) Skin and conjunctival biopsies in adrenoleukodystrophy. Acta Neuropathol (Berl) 38: 247–250
7 Montagna W (1962) The structure and function of skin, 2nd edn. Academic Press, New York, pp 320–321
8 Pinkus H, Mehregan AH (1981) A guide to dermatohistopathology, 3rd edn. Appleton-Century-Crofts, New York, p 34
9 Rupec M (1977) Zur Ultrastruktur und sauren Phosphatase-Aktivität in den Schweißdrüsen mit "clear, reticulated cytoplasm". Arch Dermatol Res 258: 193–201
10 Tsuji T, Yamamoto T (1976) Acquired generalized anhidrosis. Arch Dermatol 112: 1310–1314

Fig. 47. Secretory cells with clear cytoplasm. Different specimen to that in Fig. 46. ▷
H and E, × 400

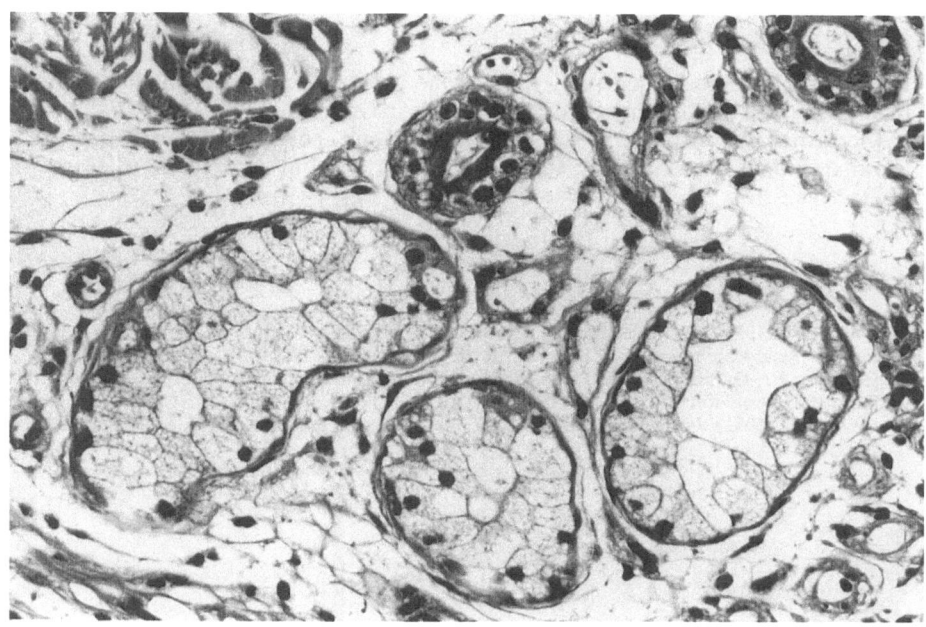

Fig. 46. The cytoplasm in the secretory cells is very clear and reticulated; the cells resemble sebaceous cells. H and E, × 400

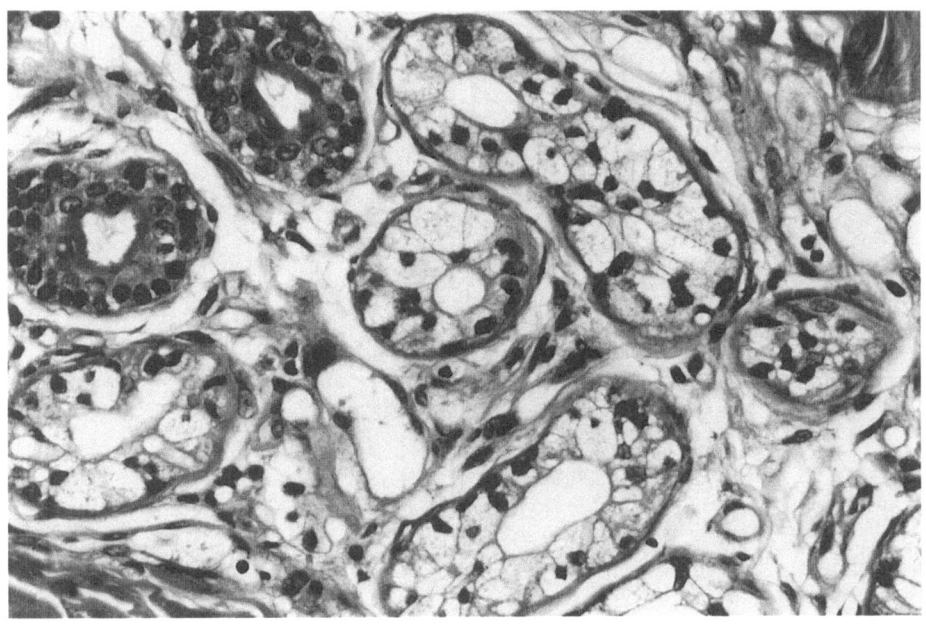

Dilatation and proliferation of sweat ducts

During pathological processes, the eccrine sweat ducts undergo dilatation and proliferation. These changes are considerable in squamous cell carcinoma [2, 10, 11, 15], keratoacanthoma [1, 3, 4, 8, 11, 13, 14], and clear cell acanthoma [5, 6, 15]. They are also evident in basal cell epithelioma [7, 8, 11, 15] and other forms of dermatosis [8, 9, 11, 12, 15].

REFERENCES

1 Andrade R (1958) Zum Verhalten der Schweißdrüsenausführungsgänge im Keratoakanthom (Molluscum pseudocarcinomatosum) (Ein kasuistischer Beitrag). Z Hautkr 24: 80–83
2 Carapeto FJ, Garcia-Perez A (1972) Adenoacanthoma: A review of 20 cases, compared with the literature. Dermatologica 145: 269–279
3 Civatte J (1982) Histopathologie cutanée, 2nd edn. Flammarion Médecine-Science, Paris, pp 314–318

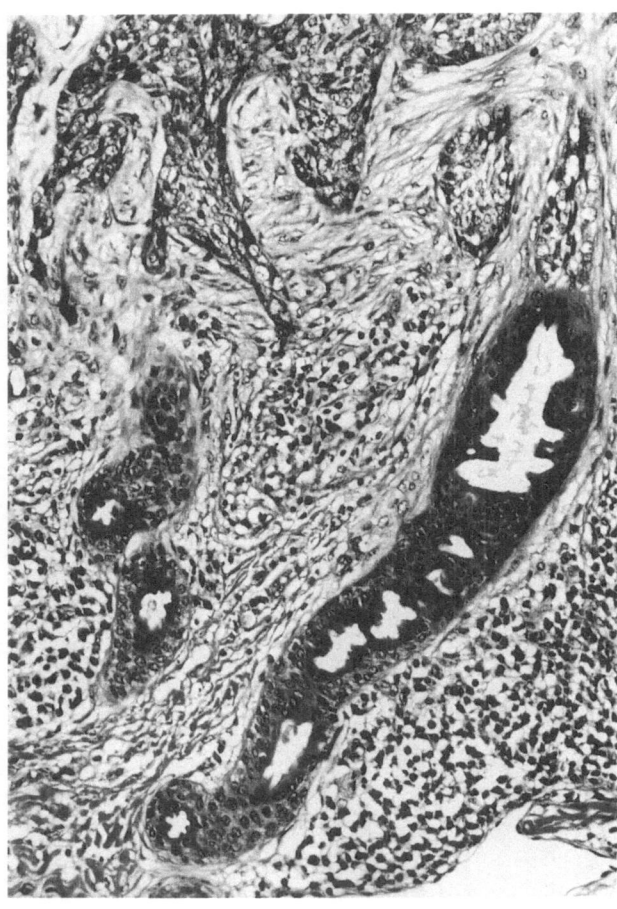

Fig. 48. Dilated sweat ducts adjoin the tumor masses of basal-cell epithelioma. Papillary projections into the lumina are seen.
H and E, × 200

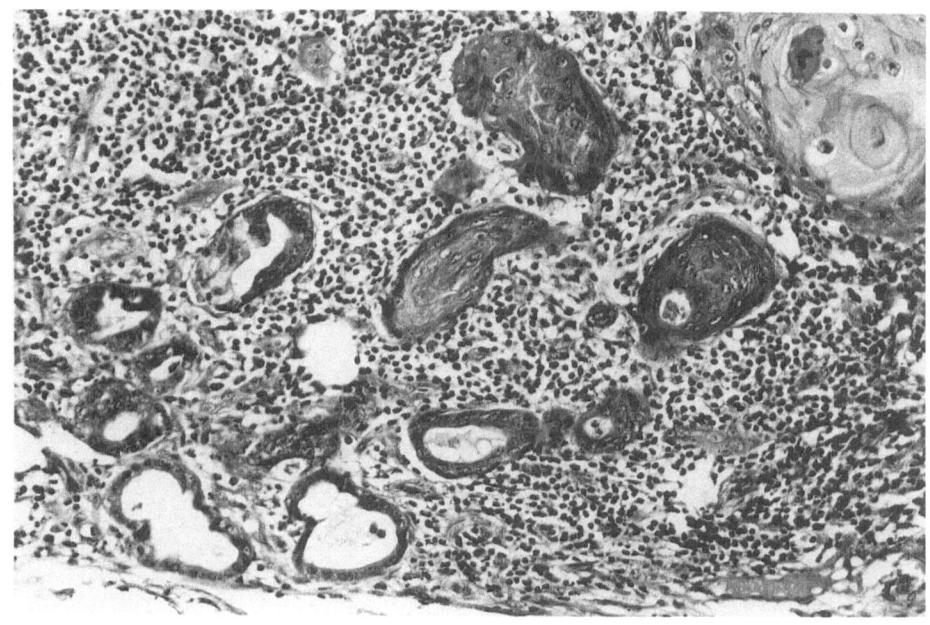

Fig. 49. Cystic dilatation and squamous metaplasia of the sweat ducts are noted at the base of the keratoacanthoma. A tumor island of the keratoacanthoma is evident in the upper right corner.
H and E, × 200

4 Civatte J (1985) Pseudo-carcinomatous hyperplasia. J Cutan Pathol 12: 214–223

5 Cramer HJ (1971) Klarzellenakanthom (Degos) mit syringomatösen und naevus-sebaceus-artigen Anteilen. Dermatologica 143: 265–270

6 Degos R, Civatte J (1970) Clear-cell acanthoma: Experience of 8 years. Br J Dermatol 83: 248–254

7 Foot NC (1947) Adnexal carcinoma of the skin. Am J Pathol 23: 1–27

8 Freeman RG (1974) On the pathogenesis of pseudoepitheliomatous hyperplasia. J Cutan Pathol 1: 231–237

9 King DT, Barr RJ (1979) Syringometaplasia: Mucinous and squamous variants. J Cutan Pathol 6: 284–291

10 Lever WF, Schaumburg-Lever G (1983) Histopathology of the skin, 6th edn. Lippincott, Philadelphia, pp 503–504

11 Mehregan AH (1981) Proliferation of sweat ducts in certain diseases of the skin. Am J Dermatopathol 3: 27–31

12 Pinkus H, Mehregan AH (1981) A guide to dermatohistopathology, 3rd edn. Appleton-Century-Crofts, New York, p 34

13 Santa Cruz DJ, Clausen K (1977) Atypical sweat duct hyperplasia accompanying keratoacanthoma. Dermatologica 154: 156–160

14 Uyeno K, Ohmi T, Wakashin K, Azuma C, Kato R, Takahashi H (1976) A clinico-histological study of keratoacanthoma in Japan with special reference to radiotherapy. In: Toda K, Ishibashi Y, Hori Y, Morikawa F (eds) Biology and disease of the hair. University of Tokyo Press, Tokyo, pp 337–357

15 Wilson Jones E, Wells GC (1966) Degos' acanthoma (Acanthome à cellules claires): A clinical and histological report of nine cases. Arch Dermatol 94: 286–294

Abnormalities of eccrine sweat ducts

REFERENCES

1 Giacometti L, Machida H (1965) Histology and cytochemistry of human skin: XXV. Common abnormalities in the eccrine sweat glands of man. Arch Dermatol 91: 73–74
2 Holyoke JB, Lobitz WC Jr (1952) Histologic variations in the structure of human eccrine sweat glands. J Invest Dermatol 18: 147–167
3 Mehregan AH (1977) Structural abnormalities of eccrine sweat ducts. J Cutan Pathol 4: 38–40
4 Mehregan AH (1981) Proliferation of sweat ducts in certain diseases of the skin. Am J Dermatopathol 3: 27–31
5 Spearman RIC (1968) Branched eccrine sweat glands in normal human skin. Nature 219: 84–85

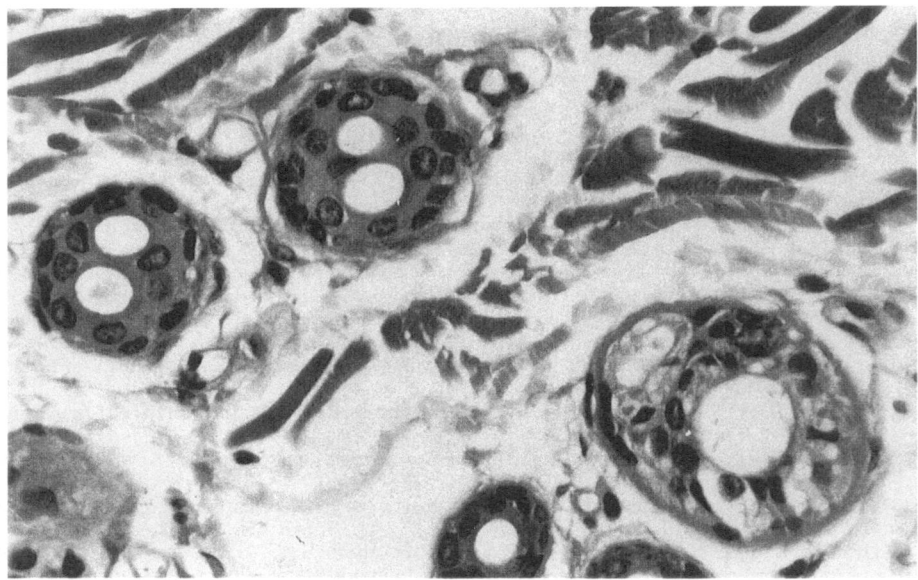

Fig. 50. Joined eccrine sweat ducts sharing a part of each cuticle are seen in two places. H and E, × 640

Fig. 51. This longitudinal
section of eccrine sweat ducts
shows a similar change
(*arrows*). The lower part of
the ducts is branching.
H and E, × 200

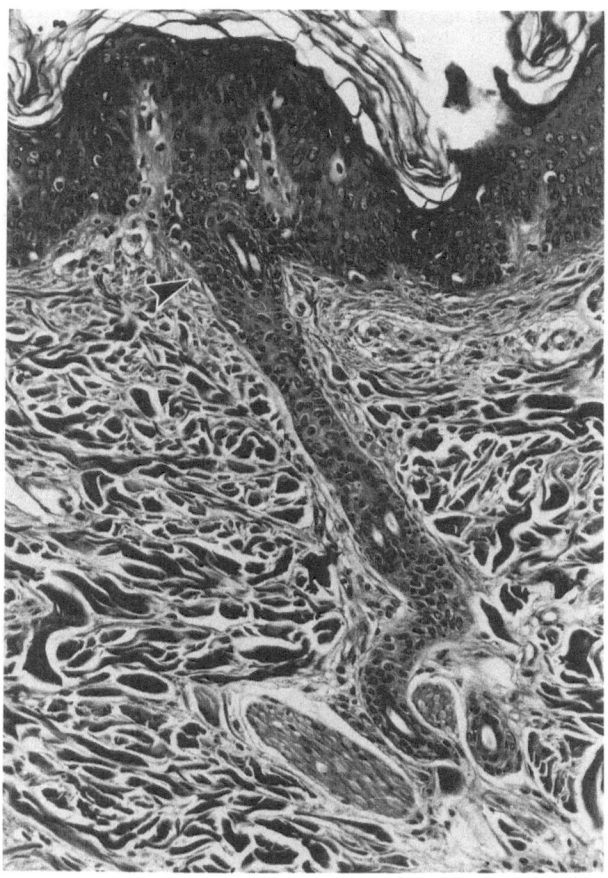

Hair follicles and sweat ducts in solar keratosis

Since the hair follicle and the eccrine sweat duct are biologically different to the epidermis, in solar keratosis they are seen to stand out clearly from the dysplastic epidermis.

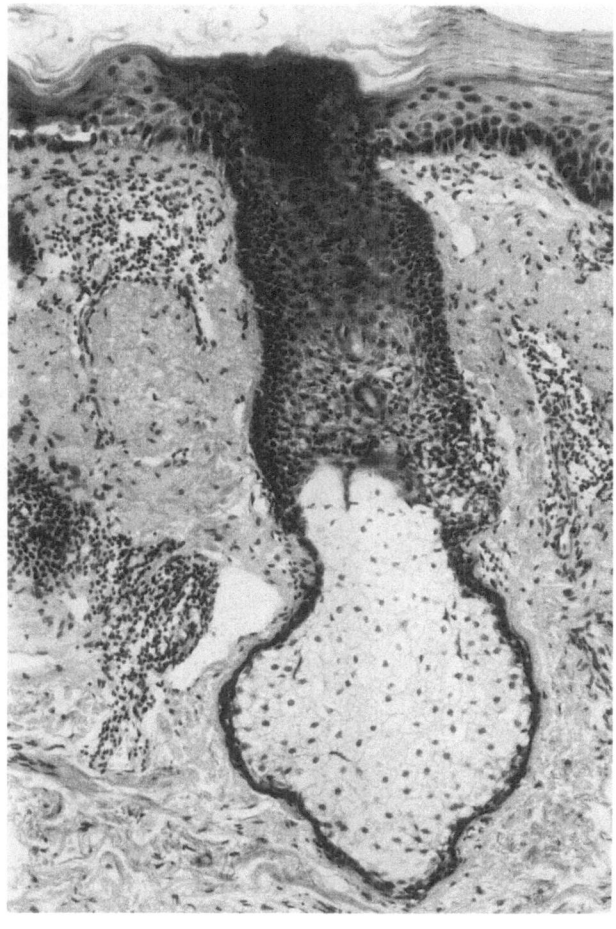

Fig. 52. A hair follicle in solar keratosis.
H and E, × 160

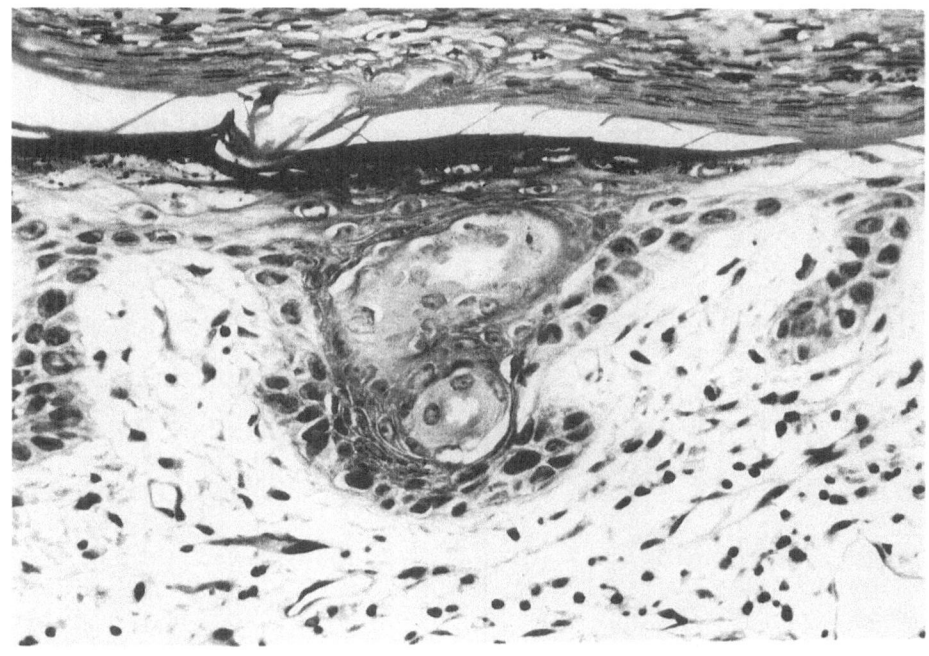

Fig. 53. A sweat duct in solar keratosis.
H and E, × 400

REFERENCES

1 Freudenthal W (1926) Verruca senilis und Keratoma senile. Arch Dermatol Syph (Berl) 152: 505–528
2 Pinkus H (1958) Keratosis senilis: A biologic concept of its pathogenesis and diagnosis based on the study of normal epidermis and 1730 seborrheic and senile keratoses. Am J Clin Pathol 29: 193–207

Tumors of the Adnexa

CYSTS

Trichilemmal cyst (Pinkus)

Trichilemmal cysts occur most frequently on the scalp. Histologically, the cyst shows the same keratinization as that of the isthmus zone of the anagen hair follicle (Figs. 18, 19) or trichilemmal sac of the catagen and telogen hair (Fig. 26). In some cases, both epidermoid and trichilemmal keratinization patterns are seen in a cyst. Such cysts were termed "hybrid cysts" by Brownstein [1].

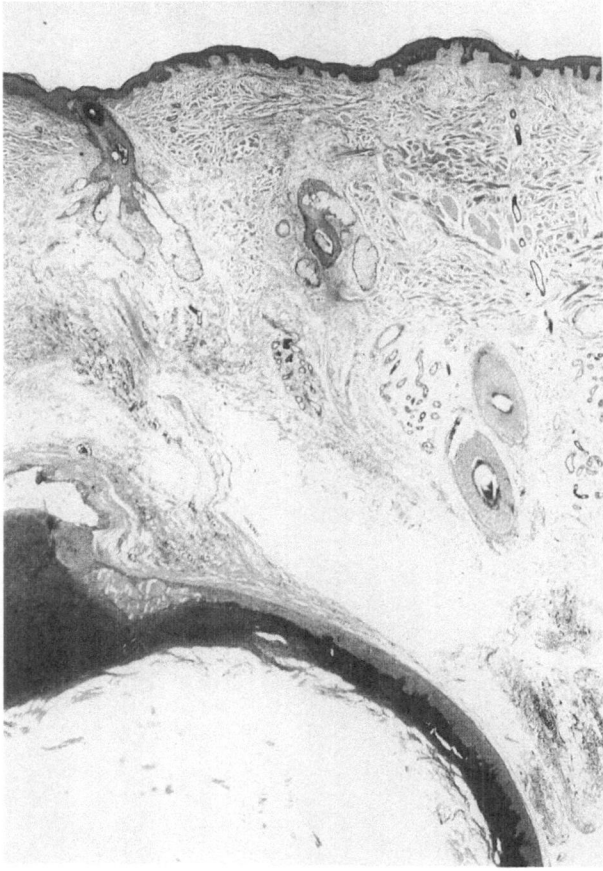

Fig. 54. The upper part of the cyst.
H and E, × 20

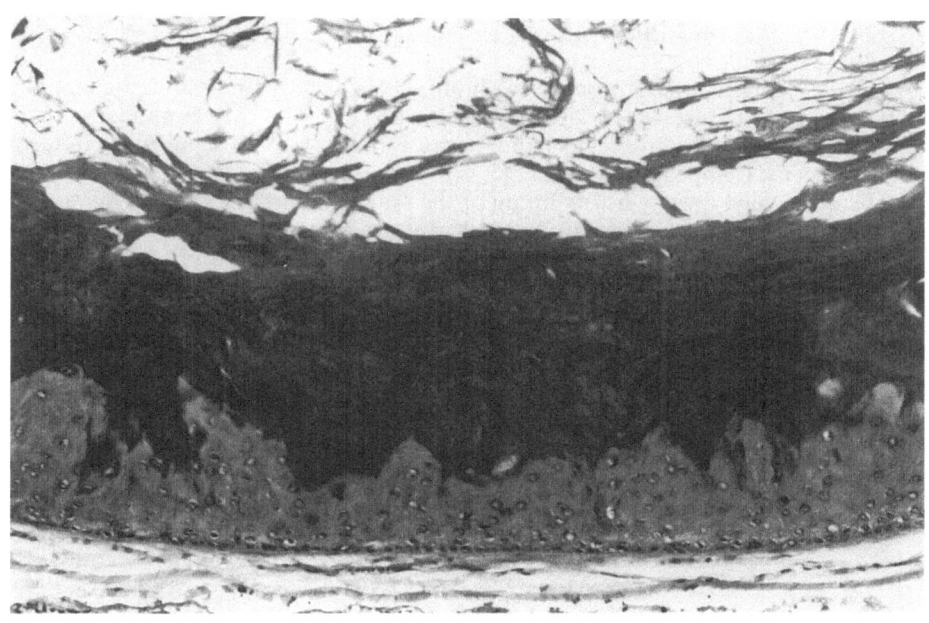

Fig. 55. Bulky cells of the cyst wall are irregularly protruding into the cystic lumen. They change abruptly into a dense homogenous keratin material without the formation of keratohyaline granules. H and E, × 160

REFERENCES

1 Brownstein MH (1983) Hybrid cyst: A combined epidermoid and trichilemmal cyst. J Am Acad Dermatol 9: 872–875
2 Kimura S (1978) Trichilemmal cysts: Ultrastructural similarities to the trichilemmal sac. Dermatologica 157: 164–170
3 Leppard BJ, Sanderson KV (1976) The natural history of trichilemmal cysts. Br J Dermatol 94: 379–390
4 Leppard BJ, Sanderson KV, Wells RS (1977) Hereditary trichilemmal cysts: Hereditary pilar cysts. Clin Exp Dermatol 2: 23–32
5 Pinkus H (1969) "Sebaceous cysts" are trichilemmal cysts. Arch Dermatol 99: 544–555

Steatocystoma multiplex

As the name indicates, steatocystoma multiplex is usually found in large numbers, but solitary structures have also been described [2]. The cyst contains a creamy substance, often including vellus hairs. Because steatocystoma is under the influence of androgens, it appears at puberty [5, 6].

Histologically, a wavy horny lining of the cyst wall without keratohyaline granules is a characteristic of steatocystoma. In addition, sebaceous glands are seen within or close to the cyst wall. According to Plewing et al., only one vellus hair follicle opens into the cyst [5, 6]. This follicle, as described by Kligman and Kirschbaum [4], seems to lie close to and parallel to the cyst wall and undergoes the hair-cyclic activity in this position.

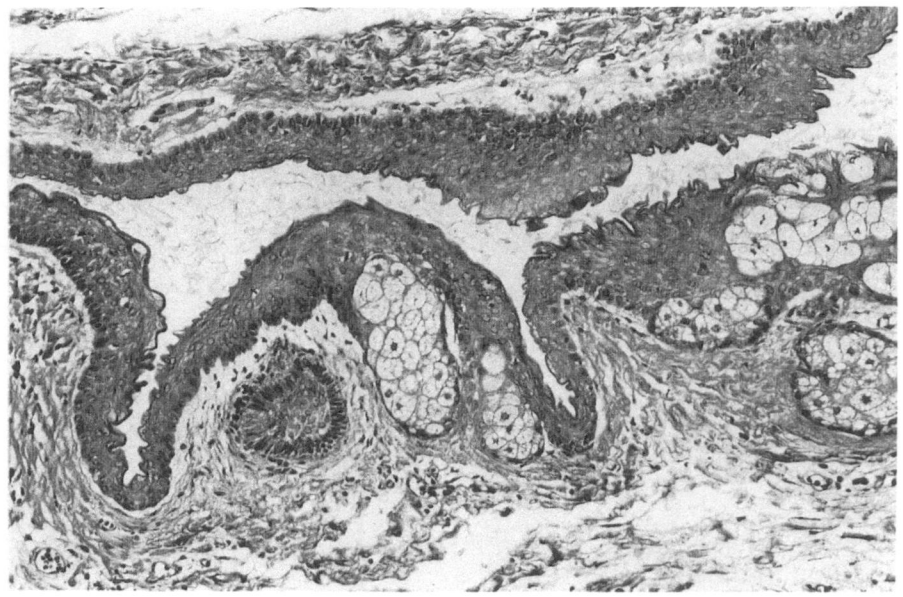

Fig. 56 The matrix-papilla complex of the hair follicle belonging to the cyst is seen embedded in the same fine fibrous sheath as that around the sebaceous glands.
H and E, × 160

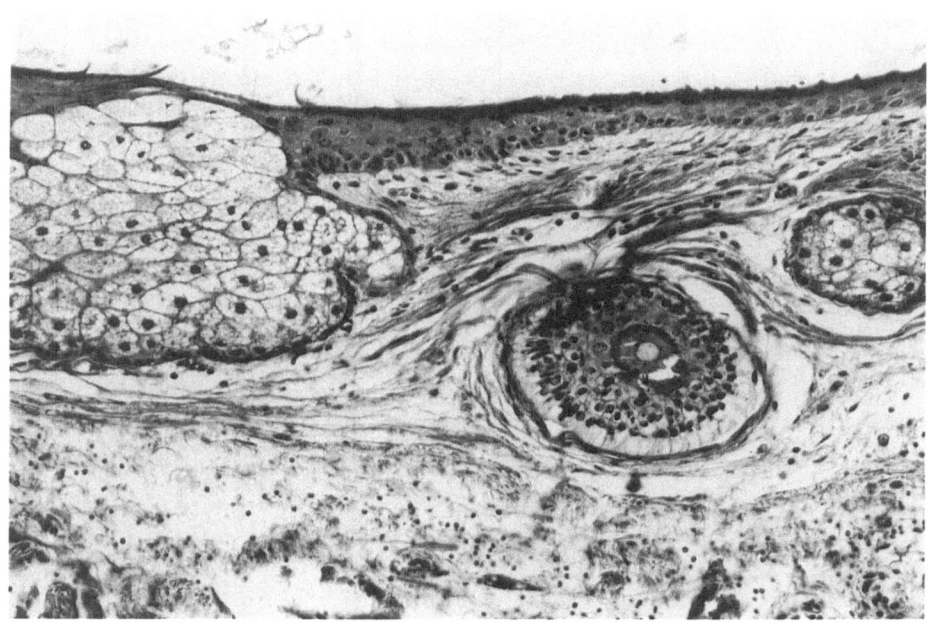

Fig. 57. The anagen hair follicle belonging to the cyst is enclosed in a fine fibrous sheath around the cyst.
H and E, × 200

REFERENCES

1 Bode U, Plewig G (1980) Klassifikation follikulärer Zysten: Epidermalzysten einschließlich Sebocys-tomatosis Günther, Steatocystoma multiplex und Trichilemmalzysten. Hautarzt 31: 1–9
2 Brownstein MH (1982) Steatocystoma simplex: A solitary steatocystoma. Arch Dermatol 118: 409–411
3 Kimura S (1981) An ultrastructural study of steatocystoma multiplex and the normal pilosebaceous apparatus. J Dermatol (Tokyo) 8: 459–465
4 Kligman AM, Kirschbaum JD (1964) Steatocystoma multiplex: A dermoid tumor. J Invest Dermatol 42: 383–387
5 Plewig G, Wolff HH, Braun-Falco O (1977) Steatocystoma multiplex—Klinik, Histologie, Elek-tronenmikroskopie, Autoradiographie. Hautarzt 28 (Suppl II): 353–354
6 Plewig G, Wolff HH, Braun-Falco O (1982) Steatocystoma multiplex: Anatomic reevaluation, electron microscopy, and autoradiography. Arch Dermatol Res 272: 363–380
7 Taniguchi S, Hirone T (1981) Light and electron microscopic studies of steatocystoma multiplex. In: Orfanos CE, Montagna W, Stüttgen G (eds) Hair research: Status and future aspects. Springer, Berlin, pp 379–384

Dermoid cyst

Dermoid cysts are present at birth. The cyst is found mostly on the head and occasionally on the neck. Since it arises from the inclusion of cutaneous tissues along the lines of embryonic closure, the structure of the cyst wall is the same as that of the epidermis; the cyst shows epidermoid keratinization and the cutaneous adnexa are seen to belong to the cyst wall.

REFERENCES

1 Brownstein MH, Helwig EB (1973) Subcutaneous dermoid cysts. Arch Dermatol 107: 237–239
2 Hogan D, Wilkinson RD, Williams A (1980) Congenital anomalies of the head and neck. Int J Dermatol 19: 479–486
3 Johnson BL, Broughton WL (1979) Ocular dermoid. J Dermatol (Tokyo) 6: 371–373
4 Kondo M (1972) Pathology of skin structures in dermoid cyst of ovary. Jpn J Dermatol Ser B 82: 58–71
5 Pollard ZF, Harley RD, Calhoun J (1976) Dermoid cysts in children. Pediatrics 57: 379–382

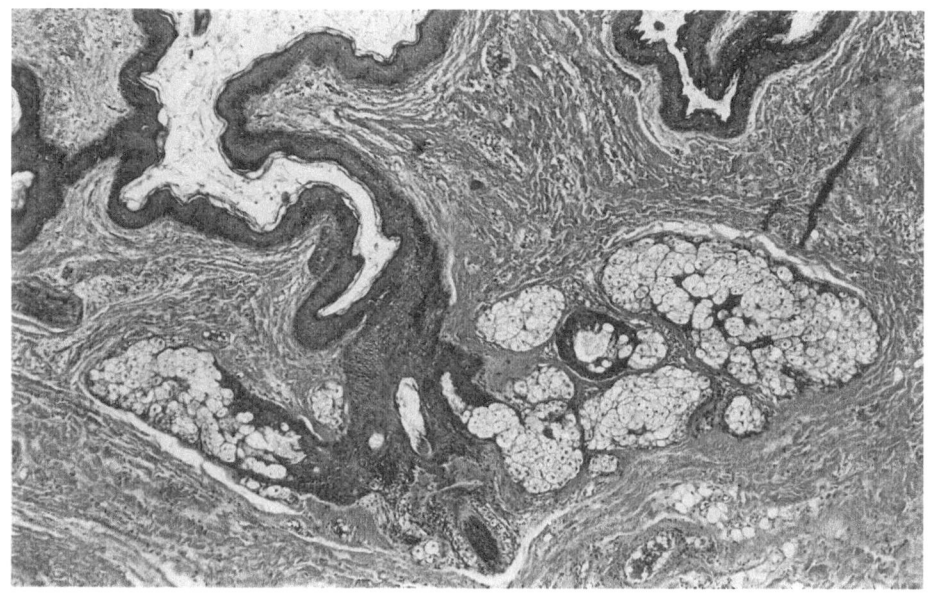

Fig. 58. A hair follicle is seen opening into the epidermoid cyst wall.
H and E, × 64

FOLLICULAR TUMORS

Inverted follicular keratosis (Helwig), porome folliculaire (Duperrat and Mascaro)

Inverted follicular keratosis is a verrucous nodule; the majority of the nodules are found on the face. The question as to whether this tumor is of follicular origin is still unsettled [1].

REFERENCES

1 Controversies in dermatopathology (1983) Am J Dermatopathol 5: 427–475
2 Duperrat B, Mascaro JM (1963) Une tumeur bénigne développée aux dépens de l'acrotrichium ou partie intraépidermique du follicule pilaire: porome folliculaire (acanthome folliculaire intraépidermique; acrotrichoma). Dermatologica 126: 291–310
3 Mehregan AH (1964) Inverted follicular keratosis. Arch Dermatol 89: 229–235
4 Mehregan AH, Nadji M (1984) Inverted follicular keratosis and *verruca vulgaris*: An investigation for the papillomavirus common antigen. J Cutan Pathol 11: 99–102
5 Sim-Davis D, Marks R, Wilson-Jones E (1976) The inverted follicular keratosis: A surprising variant of seborrheic wart. Acta Derm Venereol (Stockh) 56: 337–344

Fig. 60. At the periphery of the lobule, basaloid cells are seen. The inward cells are squamoid and ▷ numerous whorls of squamous cells (squamous eddies) are noted.
H and E, × 160

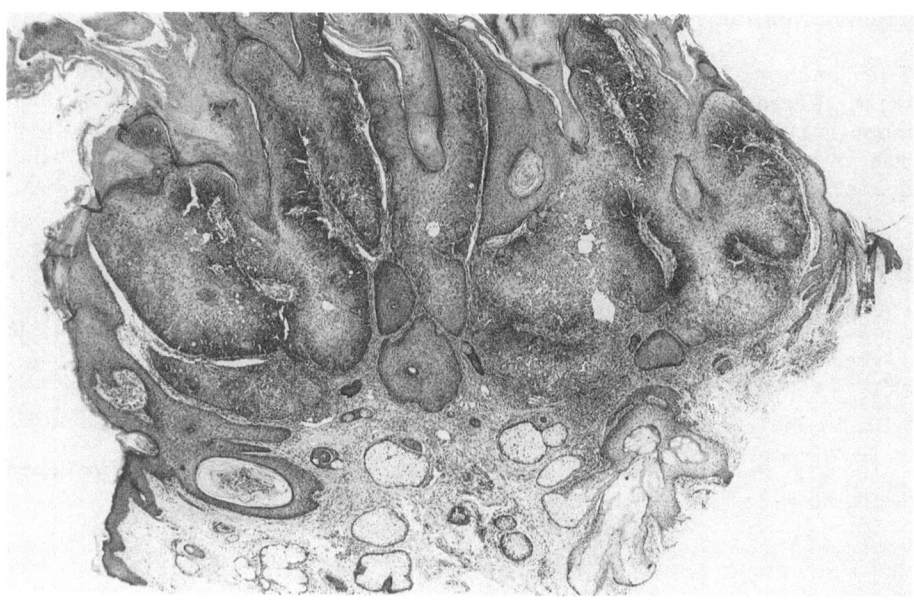

Fig. 59. Fingerlike epithelial lobules are irregularly extending downward from the surface epidermis. H and E, ×20

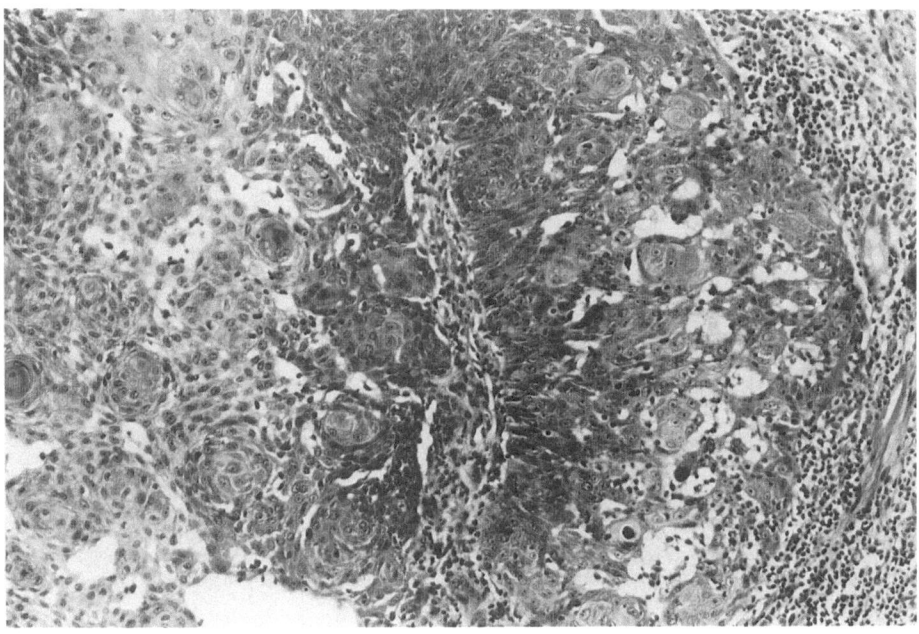

Trichilemmoma

Trichilemmoma has been regarded as a tumor differentiating toward the outer root sheath. Recently, the view was expressed by Ackerman and Wade that trichilemmoma is a verruca vulgaris with trichilemmal differentiation [1]. The tumor cells are clear owing to the abundance of glycogen. Multiple trichilemmomas in Cowden's disease are well documented [5].

REFERENCES

1 Ackerman AB, Wade TR (1980) Tricholemmoma. Am J Dermatopathol 2: 207–224
2 Brownstein MH, Shapiro L (1973) Trichilemmoma: Analysis of 40 new cases. Arch Dermatol 107: 866–869
3 Chan P, White SW, Pierson DL, Rodman OG (1979) Trichilemmoma. J Dermatol Surg Oncol 5: 58–59
4 Headington JT, French AJ (1962) Primary neoplasms of the hair follicle: Histogenesis and classification. Arch Dermatol 86: 430–441
5 Starink TM, Meijer CJLM, Brownstein MH (1985) The cutaneous pathology of Cowden's disease: new findings. J Cutan Pathol 12: 83–93

Fig. 62. The tumor consists of glycogen-rich clear cells. At the periphery, a palisade arrangement of the ▷ tumor cells is seen. This is a comparable picture to the lower portion of the outer root sheath of the anagen hair follicle (Fig. 17).
H and E, × 320

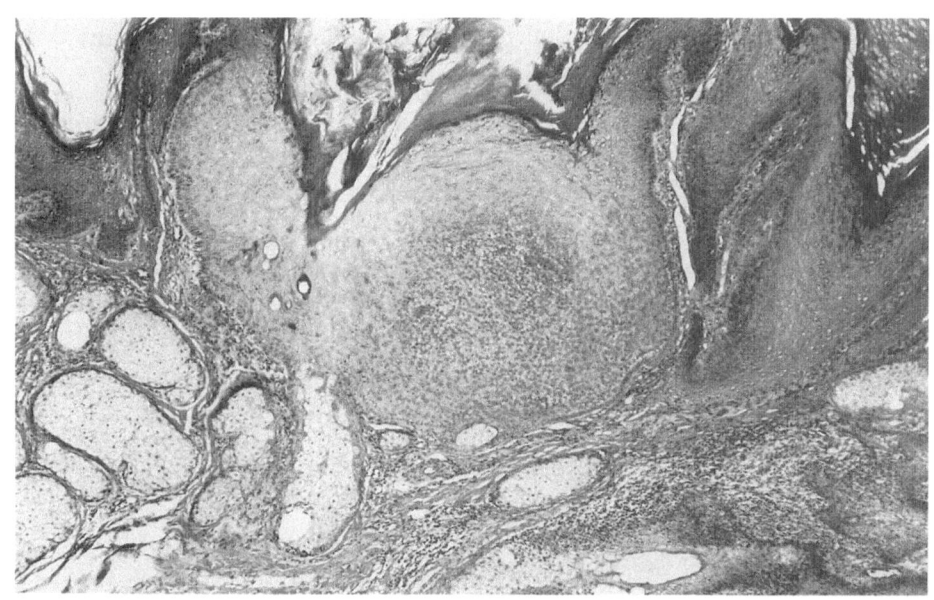

Fig. 61. This is a trichilemmoma found in nevus sebaceus.
H and E, × 64

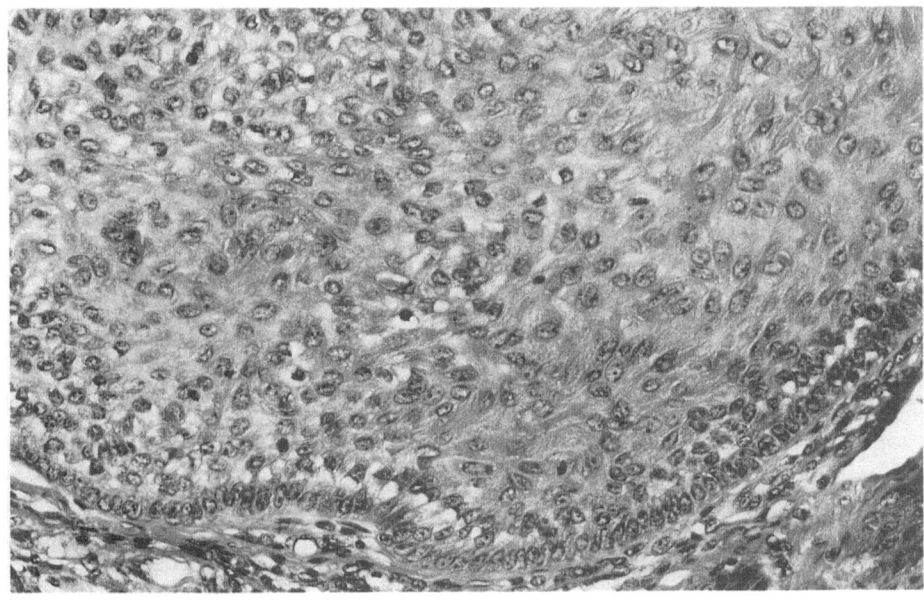

Calcifying epithelioma (Malherbe and Chenantais), pilomatricoma

Calcifying epithelioma is a firm intradermal nodule covered with normal skin. It is regarded as a tumor of the hair matrix [4,5] and the name pilomatricoma is preferable to calcifying epithelioma. The most frequent sites are the face and arms. Since pilomatricoma is occasionally pigmented, this should be kept in mind in the differential diagnosis of pigmented tumors [2,10]. Rarely, cases of giant type are reported [9]. Some pilomatricomas develop on an epidermal cyst [6]. Multiple familial pilomatricomas are regarded as a cutaneous marker of myotonic dystrophy [3]. In Japan, cases of bulla-like pilomatricoma are reported [8]; they correspond to Malherbe's tumors, showing the anetodermic changes described by Moulin et al.[7].

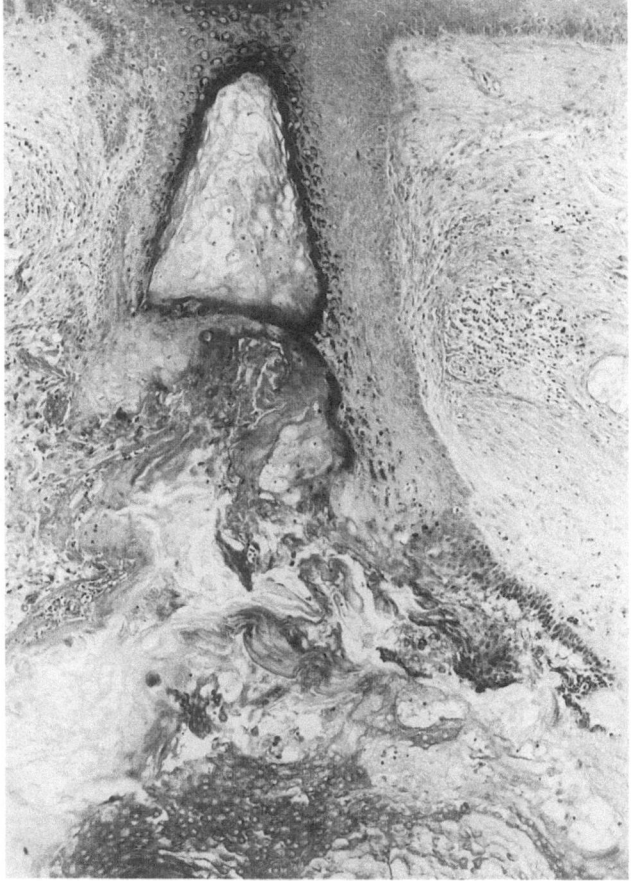

Fig. 63. In this case, in continuity with the epithelium of follicular infundibulum, tumor masses are proliferating downward in the dermis. Two kinds of tumor cell are recognized—basophilic and shadow cells.
H and E, × 100

Fig. 64. Basophilic cells
are changing into
shadow cells.
H and E, × 200

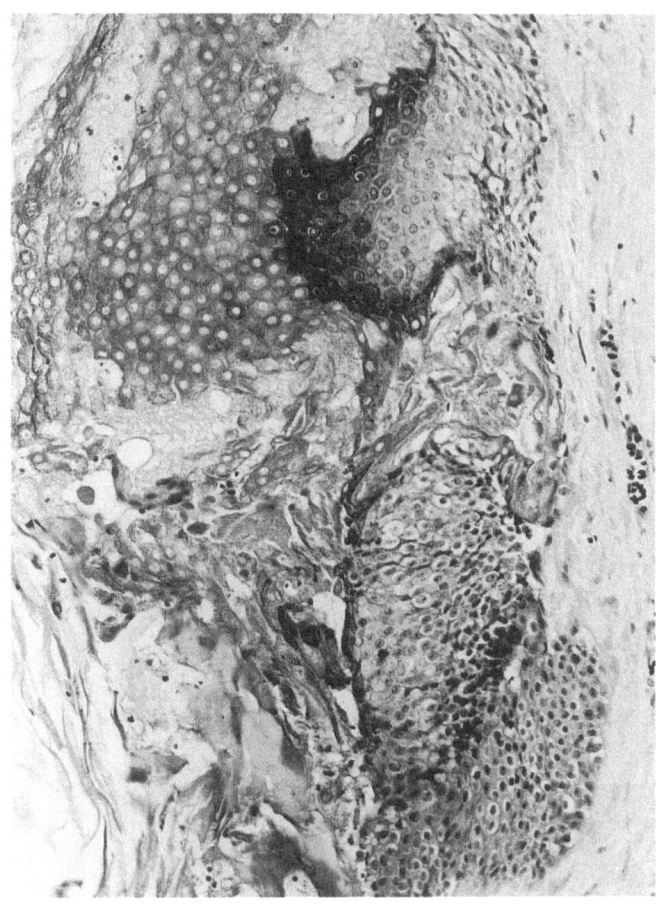

REFERENCES

1 Aso M, Shimao S, Takahashi K (1981) Pilomatricomas: Association with myotonic dystrophy. Dermatologica 162: 197–202
2 Bettendorf U, Boublik V (1983) Melaninhaltiges Pilomatrixom (Epithelioma calcificans Malherbe). Z Hautkr 58: 684–688
3 Delfino M, Monfrecola G, Ayala F, Suppa F, Piccirillo A (1985) Multiple familial pilomatricomas: A cutaneous marker for myotonic dystrophy. Dermatologica 170: 128–132
4 Forbis R Jr, Helwig EB (1961) Pilomatrixoma (calcifying epithelioma). Arch Dermatol 83: 606–618
5 Hashimoto K, Nelson RG, Lever WF (1966) Calcifying epithelioma of Malherbe: Histochemical and electron microscopic studies. J Invest Dermatol 46: 391–408
6 Kanitakis J, Hermier C, Chouvet B, Thivolet J (1984) Epithélioma calcifié de Malherbe à type histologique particulier. Dermatologica 168: 259–262
7 Moulin G, Bouchet B, Dos Santos G (1978) Les modifications anétodermiques du tégument au-dessus des tumeurs de Malherbe. Ann Dermatol Venereol 105: 43–47

8 Nagatani H, Akizuki M, Nin S, Miyashita A, Kobayashi K, Wakabayashi S, Kishimoto S (1984) Calcifying epithelioma showing bulla-like appearance. Acta Dermatol (Kyoto) 79: 271–279
9 Rothman D, Kendall AB, Baldi A (1976) Giant pilomatrixoma (Malherbe calcifying epithelioma). Arch Surg 111: 86–87
10 Spitz D, Fisher D, Friedman RJ, Kopf AW (1981) Pigmented pilomatricoma: A clinical simulator of malignant melanoma. J Dermatol Surg Oncol 7: 903–906
11 Zina AM, Bundino S, Torre C (1985) Gross pathology and scanning electron microscopy of pilomatricoma. J Cutan Pathol 12: 33–36

Hair follicle nevus, naevus pilo-follicularis (Hornstein and Weidner)

Histologically, numerous tiny hair follicles are seen in this papular nevus. They are mature and capable of producing hairs.

REFERENCES

1 Hornstein OP, Weidner F (1979) Tumoren der Haut. In: Doerr W, Seifert G, Uehlinger E (eds) Spezielle pathologische Anatomie: Ein Lehr-und Nachschlagewerk, 2nd edn, vol. 7, part 2. Springer, Berlin, p 149
2 Pinkus H, Mehregan AH (1981) A guide to dermatohistopathology, 3rd edn. Appleton-Century-Crofts, New York, pp 423–424
3 Pippione M, Aloi F, Depaoli MA (1984) Hair-follicle nevus. Am J Dermatopathol 6: 245–247

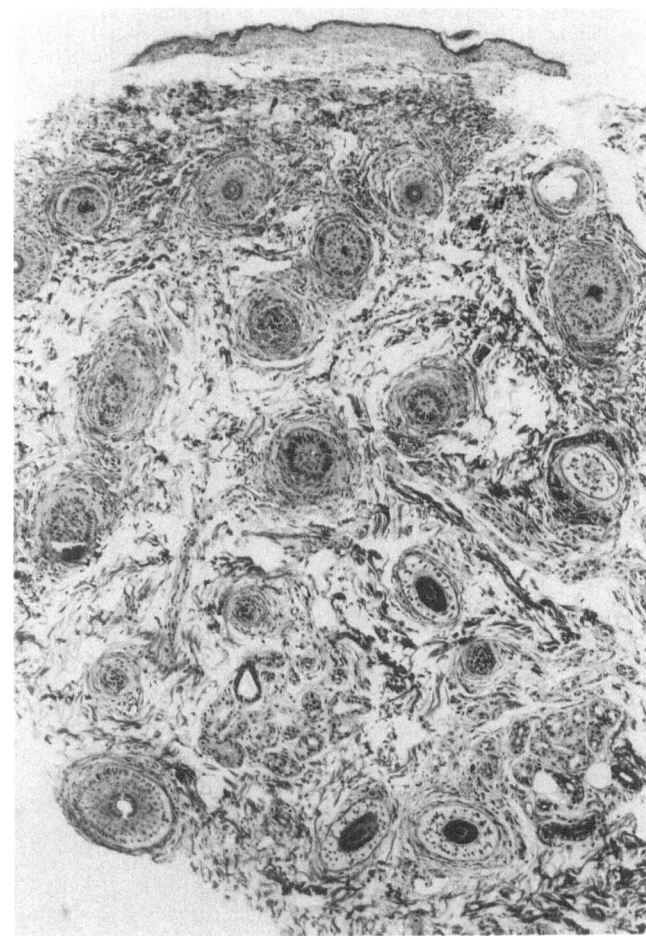

Fig. 65. A large number of follicles of the vellus hair type are seen in a papule. In this case, a few nevus cells are noted around some of the follicles. H and E, × 80

Trichofolliculoma (Miescher)

Trichofolliculoma occurs usually on the face as a dome-shaped nodule. As expressed by the French name *naevus annexiel en soie floche* [1], this tumor has a central pore, from which a tuft of white hairs like wool or floss silk (*soie floche*) is seen to emerge. Sebaceous trichofolliculoma, a variant of this tumor, is also recognized [5,7].

REFERENCES

1 Duperrat B, Mascaro JM, Lambergeon S (1964) Naevus annexiel en "soie floche": tricho-folliculome de Miescher. Bull Soc Fr Dermatol Syph 71: 318–320
2 Hidano A (1963) Trichofolliculome. Jpn J Dermatol Ser B 73: 231–232
3 Ishikawa K (1981) Trichofolliculoma and trichoblastic fibroma. In: Orfanos CE, Montagna W, Stüttgen G (eds) Hair research: Status and future aspects. Springer, Berlin, pp 375–378
4 Miescher G (1944) Un cas de trichofolliculome. Dermatologica 89: 193–194
5 Mohri S (1981) Pilar acanthoma: A combination of inverted follicular keratosis and sebaceous trichofolliculoma. J Dermatol (Tokyo) 8: 479–481
6 Pinkus H, Sutton RL Jr (1965) Trichofolliculoma. Arch Dermatol 91: 46–49
7 Plewig G (1980) Sebaceous trichofolliculoma. J Cutan Pathol 7: 394–403
8 Steffen C, Leaming DV (1982) Trichofolliculoma of the upper eyelid. Cutis 30: 343–345

Fig. 66. From a central dilated hair follicle, numerous tiny hair follicles are seen to radiate. Because each of these follicles produces white hairs, the hairs converge into the central follicle; here, they are twisted and emerge on the surface of the nodule.
H and E, × 40
(from Ishikawa [3])

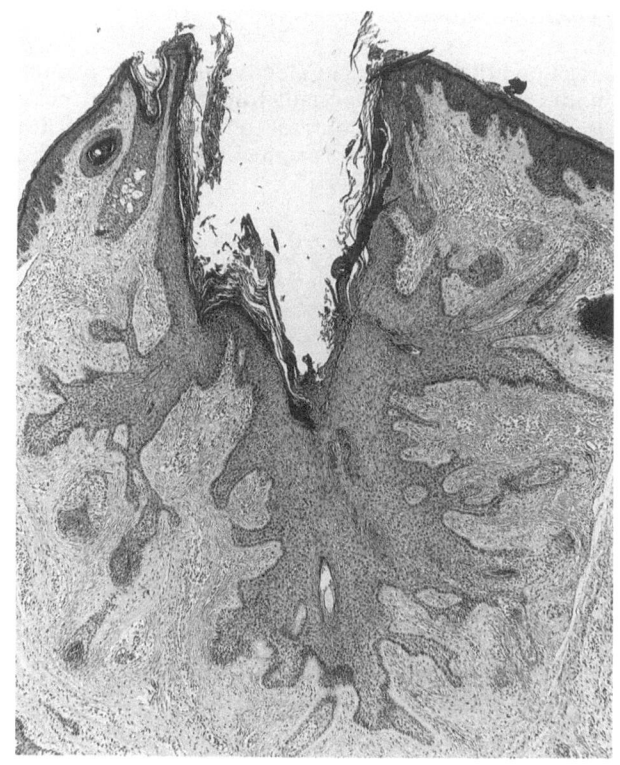

Trichoepithelioma

Trichoepitheliomas occur chiefly on the face as multiple skin-colored papules and nodules; they are occasionally found on the buttocks [8]. Solitary trichoepithelioma is also recognized. In contrast to basal cell epithelioma, the lesion does not tend to ulcerate[3]. Recently, a variant of this tumor, "desmoplastic trichoepithelioma," has been reported[1,6].

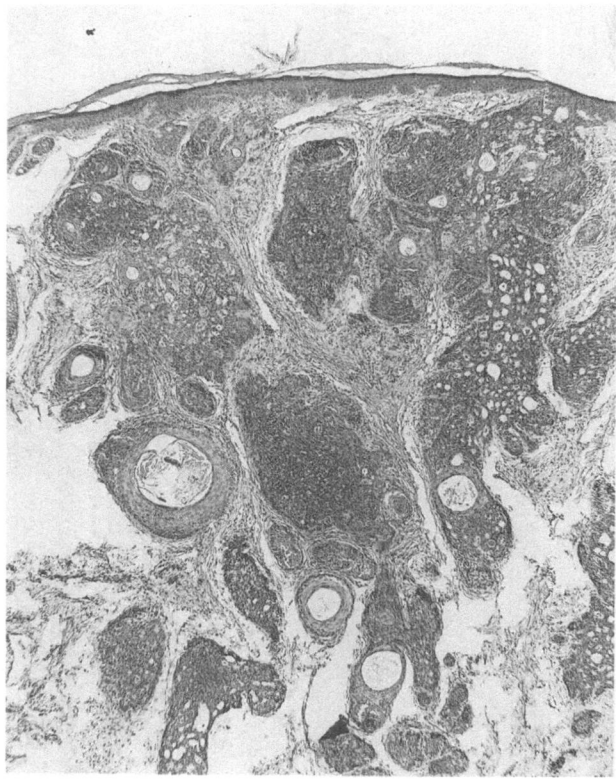

Fig. 67. Numerous tumor islands composed of basaloid cells, in which many horn cysts are seen.
H and E, ×46

80

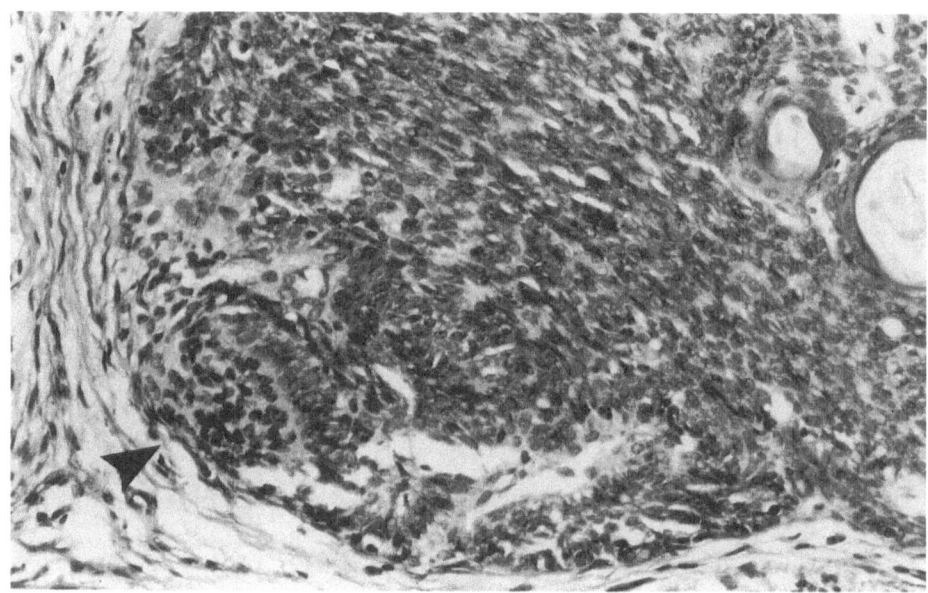

Fig. 68. On close examination, dermal papilla cell-like cells are in many places seen massed around the tumor islands, resembling an abortive hair matrix and papilla (*arrow*).
H and E, × 320

REFERENCES

1 Brownstein MH, Shapiro L (1977) Desmoplastic trichoepithelioma. Cancer 40: 2979–2986
2 Hirone T, Eryu Y, Otsuki N, Fukushiro R (1976) Light and electron microscopic studies of trichoepithelioma papulosum multiplex. In: Toda K, Ishibashi Y, Hori Y, Morikawa F (eds) Biology and disease of the hair. University of Tokyo Press, Tokyo, pp 397–407
3 Howell JB, Anderson DE (1976) Transformation of epithelioma adenoides cysticum into multiple rodent ulcers: fact or fallacy. A historical vignette. Br J Dermatol 95: 233–242
4 Ohkohchi K, Tagami H (1985) Solitary trichoepithelioma with prominent cystic structures. J Dermatol (Tokyo) 12: 91–93
5 Ono T, Sakazaki Y, Jono M, Muto K (1982) Banded structure in solitary trichoepithelioma. Acta Derm Venereol (Stockh) 62: 68–72
6 Park CW, Kim SY, Houh W (1985) Desmoplastic trichoepithelioma. Korean J Dermatol 23: 245–247
7 Ueda K, Komori Y, Maruo M, Kusaba K (1981) Ultrastructure of trichoepithelioma papulosum multiplex. J Cutan Pathol 8: 188–198
8 Vulcan P, Vulcan V, Pais V, Grigoire M (1983) Tricho-épithéliomes multiples profus de la face, du cuir chevelu et des fesses: Recherches histologique, histochimique et ultrastructurale. Ann Dermatol Venereol 110: 625–627
9 Watanabe J (1922) Über das Cylindrom und das Epithelioma adenoides cysticum. (Ergebnisse der Untersuchung eines Falles Spieglerscher Tumoren.) Arch Dermatol Syph (Berl) 140: 208–234
10 Winkelmann RK, Diaz-Perez JL (1980) Trichoepitheliome. Hautarzt 31: 527–530

Trichogenic tumors

Trichogenic tumors are sharply circumscribed nodules appearing deep at the junction of the dermis and subcutis. In this type of tumor, the stroma induces the structure of the hair follicle from the tumor epithelium. From the state of interaction between the stroma and the epithelium, Headington divided these tumors as follows—trichoblastoma, trichoblastic fibroma, trichogenic trichoblastoma, and trichogenic myxoma [5].

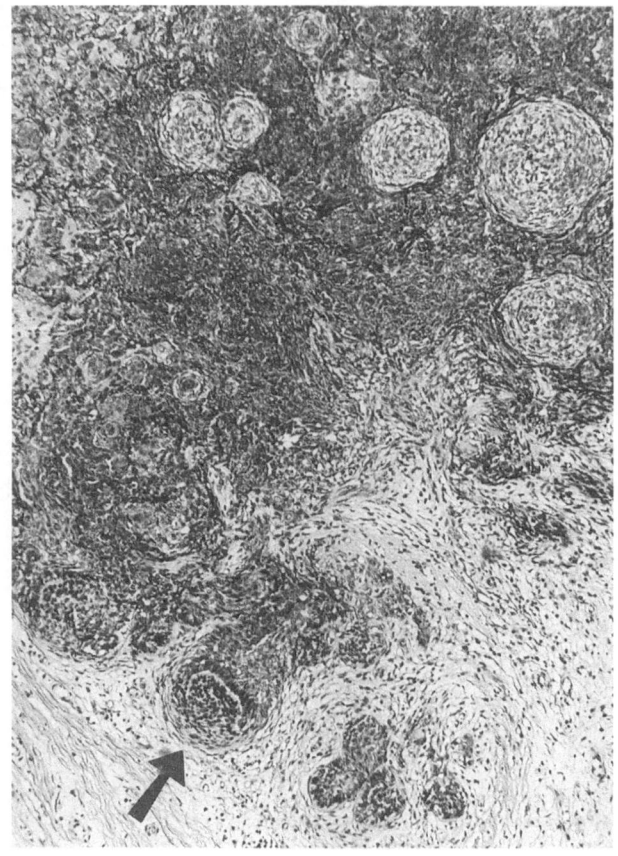

Fig. 69. Trichoblastic fibroma. The matrix-papilla portion of the hair follicle is seen arising from the tumor masses made up of basaloid cells (*arrow*).
H and E, × 78
(from Ishikawa [7])

Fig. 70. Similar picture to Fig. 69 at another site. No hair shafts are seen in these follicular structures. H and E, × 160

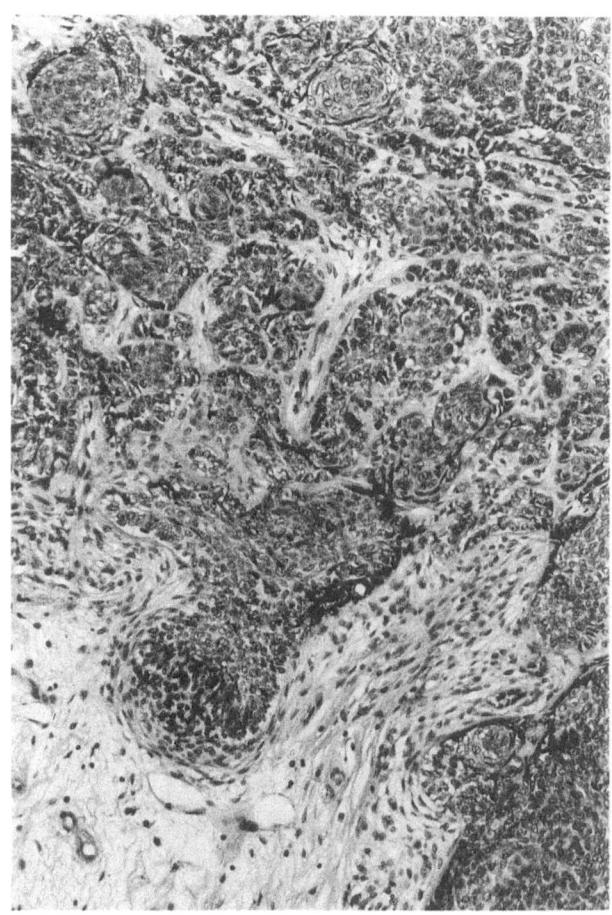

REFERENCES

1 Arata J (1976) An unusual hair follicle tumor—An intimate relative of trichogenic adnexal tumor (Headington and French). J Dermatol (Tokyo) 3: 221–229
2 Grouls V, Kupfer R (1984) Trichoblastisches Fibrom. Z Hautkr 59: 426–430
3 Headington JT, French AJ (1962) Primary neoplasms of the hair follicle: Histogenesis and classification. Arch Dermatol 86: 430–441
4 Headington JT (1970) Differentiating neoplasms of hair germ. J Clin Pathol 23: 464–471
5 Headington JT (1976) Tumors of the hair follicle: A review. Am J Pathol 85: 480–514
6 Imai S, Nitto H (1982) Trichogenes Trichoblastom. Hautarzt 33: 609–611
7 Ishikawa K (1981) Trichofolliculoma and trichoblastic fibroma In: Orfanos CE, Montagna W, Stüttgen G (eds) Hair research: Status and future aspects. Springer, Berlin, pp 375–378
8 Maruo M, Yasuno H, Kobayashi K, Nakayasu K (1982) A variant type of trichogenic trichoblastoma. Acta Dermatol (Kyoto) 77: 135–140

SEBACEOUS TUMORS

Fordyce's condition

Fordyce's condition is a well-recognized clinical manifestation of ectopic sebaceous glands observed on the vermilion border of the upper lip or on the buccal mucosa. Other ectopic sebaceous glands are seen in many parts of the body [1–3].

REFERENCES

1 Brownstein MH, Shapiro L (1977) The pilosebaceous tumors. Int J Dermatol 16: 340–352
2 Guiducci AA, Hyman AB (1962) Ectopic sebaceous glands: A review of the literature regarding their occurrence, histology and embryonic relationships. Dermatologica 125: 44–63
3 Strauss JS, Pochi PE (1968) Histology, histochemistry, and electron microscopy of sebaceous glands in man. In: Marchionini A (ed) Handbuch der Haut- und Geschlechtskrankheiten, Ergänzungswerk, vol. 1, part 1. Springer, Berlin, pp 216–219

Fig. 72. Oral mucosa with sebaceous lobules. ▷
H and E, × 64

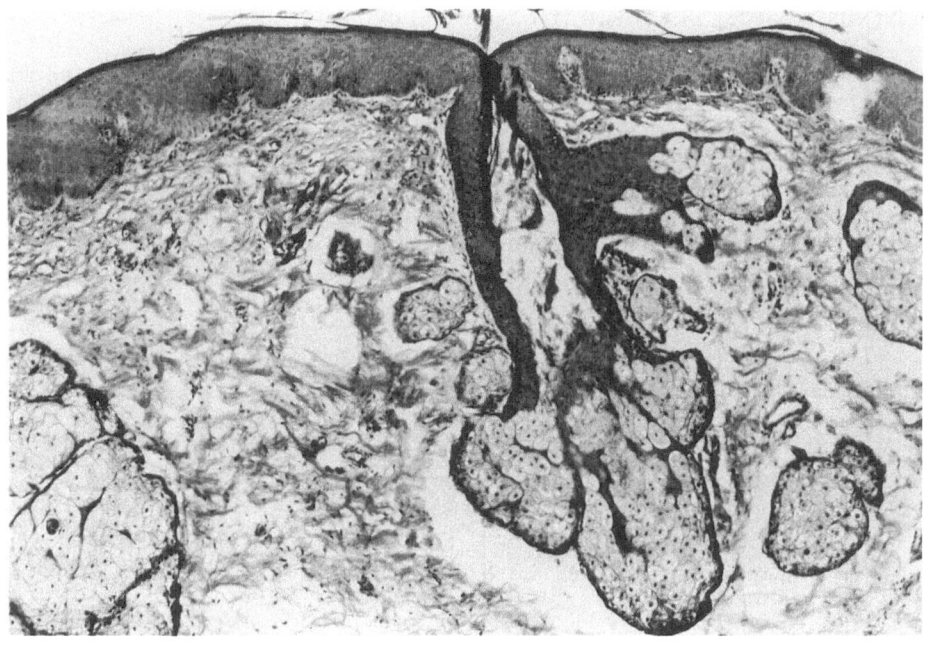

Fig. 71. Through a sebaceous duct, lobules of normal sebaceous glands are seen opening directly onto the surface epithelium of the lip.
H and E, × 80

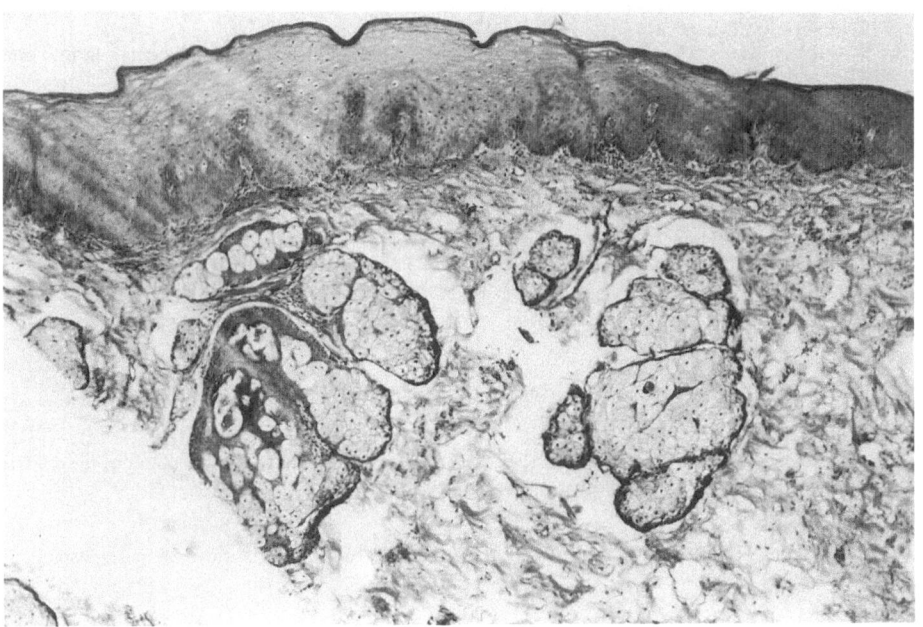

Nevus sebaceus (Jadassohn), organoid nevus

Nevus sebaceus is a congenital, hairless plaque, which occurs mostly on the scalp and face. The clinical appearance and histological findings change with age. There are three stages through the course of life: (1) The infantile stage of the Wolters type, in which the sebaceous glands are still underdeveloped; (2) the pubertal stage of the Jadassohn type, in which the sebaceous glands and the apocrine glands develop remarkably; (3) the tumor stage, in which a variety of adnexal tumors may arise in the lesion. Recently, ocular, cerebral, and skeletal abnormalities associated with this nevus (Schimmelpenning-Feuerstein-Mims syndrome) have been recognized [1, 5, 9, 11, 12].

REFERENCES

1 Bavinck JNB, van de Kamp JJP (1985) Organoid naevus phakomatosis: Schimmelpenning-Feuerstein-Mims syndrome. Br J Dermatol 113: 491–492
2 Bonvalet D, Barrandon Y, Foix Ch, Civatte J (1983) Tumeurs annexielles bénignes de survenue tardive sur naevus verruco-sébacé (Jadassohn): A propos de 7 cas. Ann Dermatol Venereol 110: 337–342
3 Coskey RJ (1982) The spectrum of organoid nevi. Cutis 29: 290–294
4 Fergin PE, Chu AC, MacDonald DM (1981) Basal cell carcinoma complicating naevus sebaceus. Clin Exp Dermatol 6: 111–115
5 Hornstein OP, Knickenberg M (1974) Zur Kenntnis des Schimmelpenning-Feuerstein-Mims-Syndroms (Organoide Naevus-Phakomatose). Arch Dermatol Forsch 250: 33–50
6 Mehregan AH, Pinkus H (1965) Life history of organoid nevi: Special reference to nevus sebaceus of Jadassohn. Arch Dermatol 91: 574–588
7 Mehregan AH (1985) Sebaceous tumors of the skin. J Cutan Pathol 12: 196–199
8 Morioka S (1985) The natural history of *nevus sebaceus*. J Cutan Pathol 12: 200–213
9 Pinkus H (1978) Organoid nevus. Mod Probl Paediatr 20: 50–57
10 Pinkus H, Mehregan AH (1981) A guide to dermatohistopathology, 3rd edn. Appleton-Century-Crofts, New York, pp 417–419
11 Sehgal VN, Ramesh V, Ghorpade A (1984) Naevus sebaceous associated with ocular dermolipoma. J Dermatol (Tokyo) 11: 97–98
12 Serpas de López RME, Hernández-Pérez E (1985) Jadassohn's sebaceous nevus. J Dermatol Surg Oncol 11: 68–72
13 Steigleder GK, Cortes AC (1971) Verhalten der Talgdrüsen im Talgdrüsennaevus während des Kindesalters. Arch Klin Exp Dermatol 239: 323–328
14 Werner A, Jadassohn J (1895) Zur Kenntniss der "systematisirten Naevi". Arch Dermatol Syph (Berl) 33: 341–408
15 Wilson Jones E, Heyl T (1970) Naevus sebaceus: A report of 140 cases with special regard to the development of secondary malignant tumours. Br J Dermatol 82: 99–117
16 Wolters M (1910) Über einen Fall von Naevus epitheliomatosus sebaceus capitis. Arch Dermatol Syph (Berl) 101: 197–208

Fig. 73. Nevus sebaceus in the stage of the Jadassohn type. Papillomatous hyperplasia of the epidermis ▷ and a large number of well-developed sebaceous glands are seen.
H and E, × 40

Fig. 74. Nevus sebaceus of a 14-year-old boy. The sebaceous glands are still underdeveloped. A ▷ rudimentary hair follicle is seen.
H and E, × 100

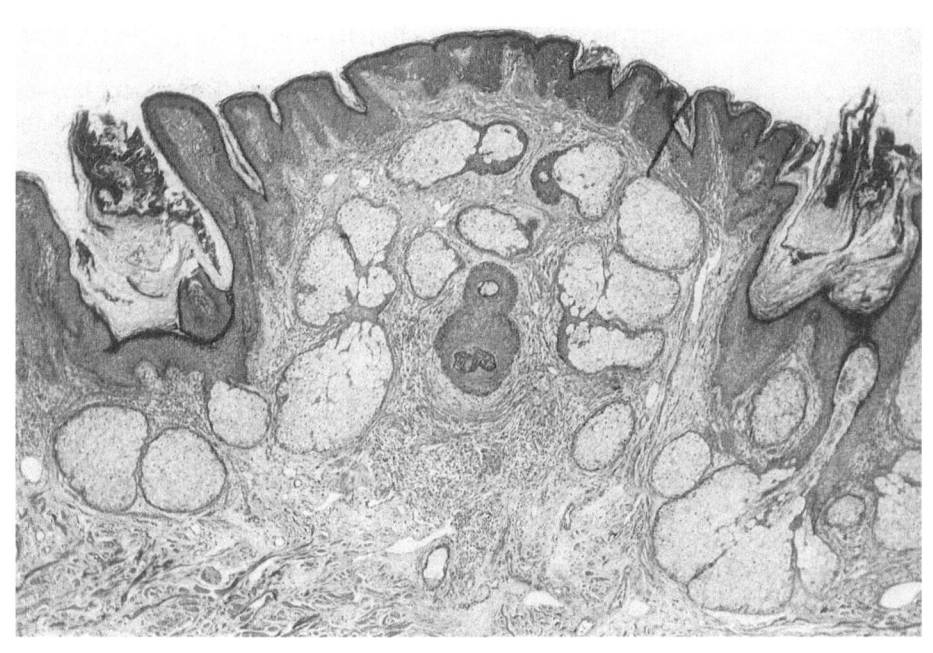

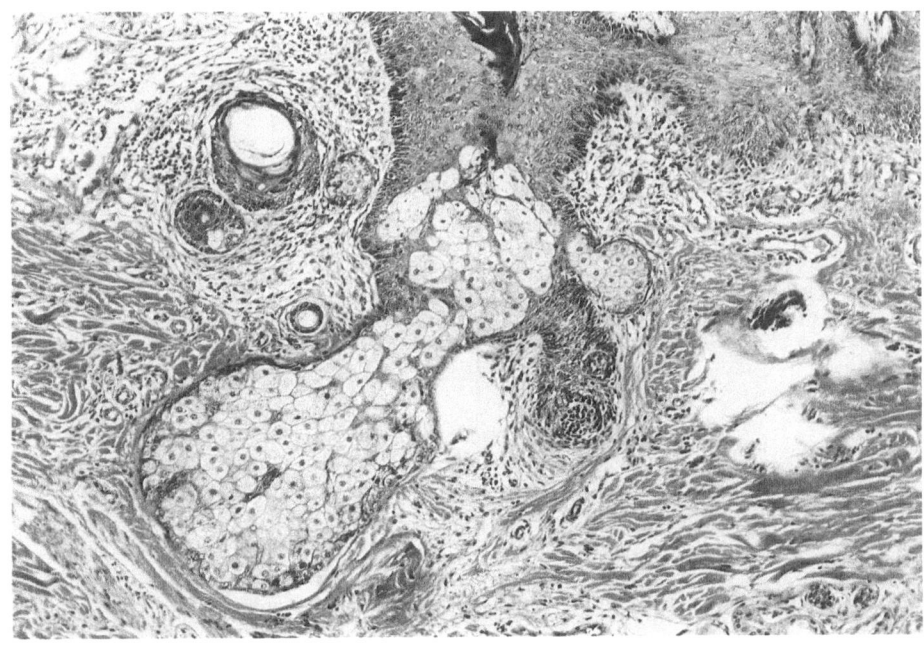

Senile sebaceous hyperplasia, sebaceous hyperplasia

Sebaceous hyperplasia occurs mostly as several, yellow, umbilicated papules on the face of persons past middle age. In this tumor, the migration of the sebocytes from the peripheral basal (germinative) cell layer of the lobule to the sebaceous duct is slower than in normal sebaceous glands [8]. Recently, new types of sebaceous hyperplasia have been reported [1, 3–7].

REFERENCES

1 Blanchet-Bardon C, Servant JM, Le Tuan B, Puissant A (1982) Hyperplasie sébacée acquise à type de cutis verticis gyrata sensible au 13-*cis*-rétinoïde. Ann Dermatol Venereol 109: 749–750
2 Braun-Falco O, Thianprasit M (1965) Über die circumscripte senile Talgdrüsenhyperplasie. Arch Klin Exp Dermatol 221: 207–231
3 Burton CS, Sawchuk WS (1985) Premature sebaceous gland hyperplasia: Successful treatment with isotretinoin. J Am Acad Dermatol 12: 182–184
4 Catalano PM, Ioannides G (1985) Areolar sebaceous hyperplasia. J Am Acad Dermatol 13: 867–868
5 De Villez RL, Roberts LC (1982) Premature sebaceous gland hyperplasia. J Am Acad Dermatol 6: 933–935
6 Dupré A, Bonafé JL, Lamon R (1980) Functional familial sebaceous hyperplasia of the face: Reverse of the Cunliffe acne-free naevus? Its inclusion among naevoid sebaceous receptor diseases. Clin Exp Dermatol 5: 203–207
7 Fernandez N, Torres A (1984) Hyperplasia of sebaceous glands in a linear pattern of papules: Report of four cases. Am J Dermatopathol 6: 237–243
8 Luderschmidt C, Plewig G (1978) Circumscribed sebaceous gland hyperplasia: Autoradiographic and histoplanimetric studies. J Invest Dermatol 70: 207–209
9 Prioleau PG, Santa Cruz DJ (1984) Sebaceous gland neoplasia. J Cutan Pathol 11: 396–414

Fig. 76. High magnification of Fig. 75. A demodex folliculorum is found in the sebaceous lobule. ▷
H and E, × 320

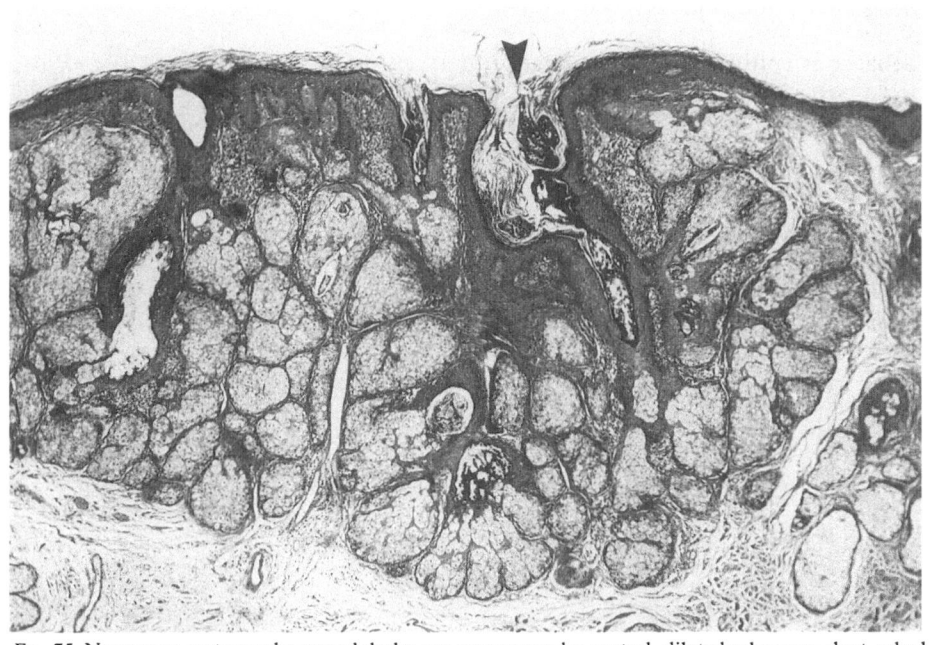

Fig. 75. Numerous mature sebaceous lobules are seen around a central, dilated sebaceous duct, which corresponds to the clinically noticeable umbilication (*arrow*).
H and E, ×40

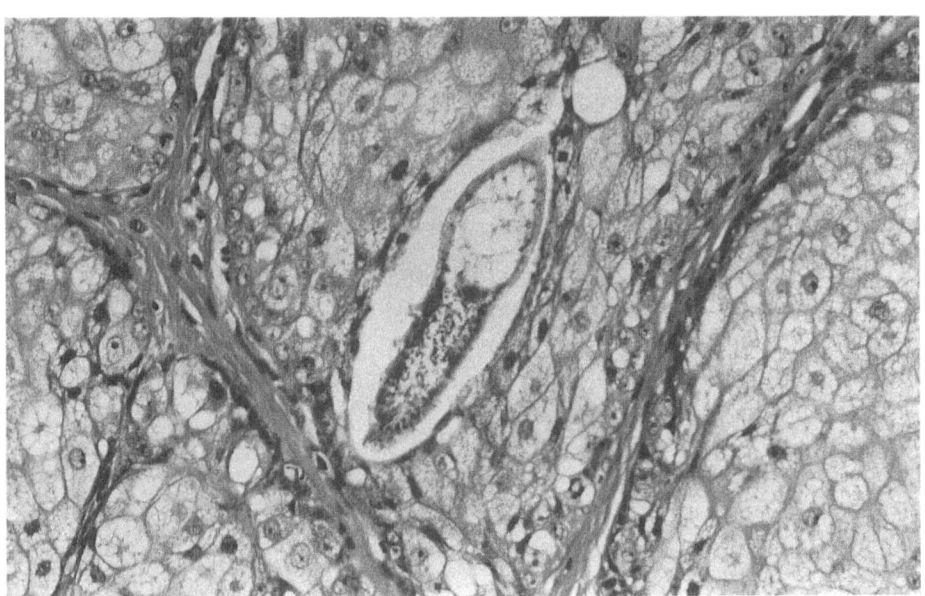

Sebaceous epithelioma

Sebaceous epithelioma occurs as a primary lesion or occasionally arises within a nevus sebaceus. Troy and Ackerman objected to the term "sebaceous epithelioma" and proposed "sebaceoma" for this type of benign adnexal neoplasm with sebaceous cell differentiation [5]. The association of sebaceous tumors including sebaceous epithelioma with multiple visceral carcinomas is now known as Torre's syndrome [1].

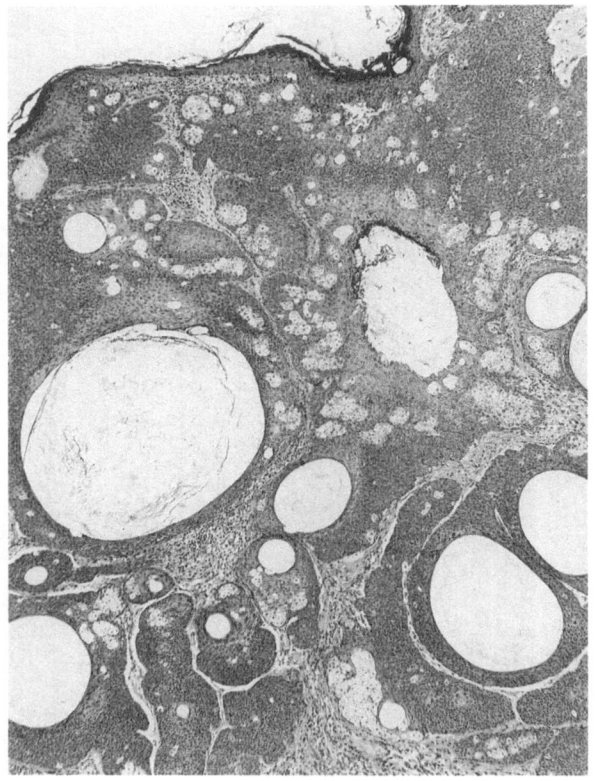

Fig. 77. The tumor consists of basaloid cells, but no peripheral palisading of the cells is noted. A large number of mature sebaceous cells, singly or in groups, are seen in the tumor masses. In addition, cysts of various size are found within them.
H and E, × 40

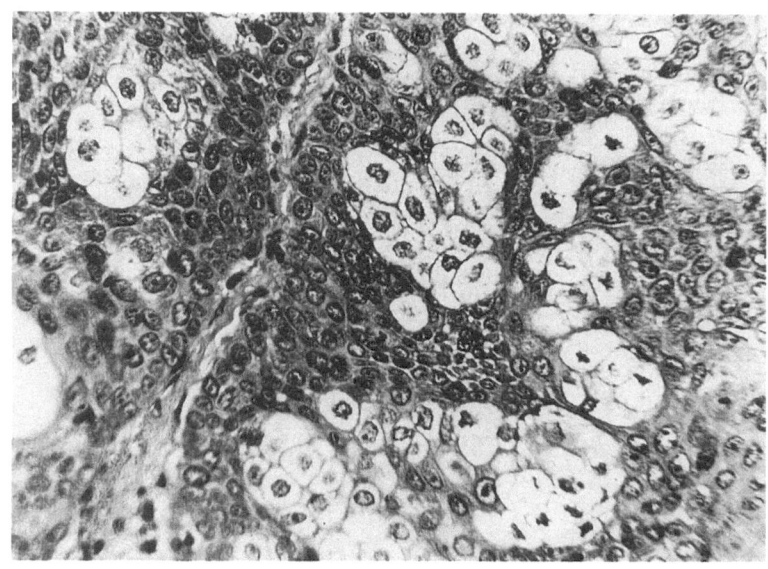

Fig. 78. High magnification of Fig. 77.
H and E, × 346

REFERENCES

1 Finan MC, Connolly SM (1984) Sebaceous gland tumors and systemic disease: A clinicopathologic analysis. Medicine (Baltimore) 63: 232–242
2 Hori M, Egami K, Maejima K, Nishimoto K (1978) Electron microscopic study of sebaceous epithelioma. J Dermatol (Tokyo) 5: 139–147
3 Niizuma K (1977) An electron microscopic study of sebaceous epithelioma: A case report with two new observations on lipid droplet formation. Dermatologica 154: 98–106
4 Rulon DB, Helwig EB (1974) Cutaneous sebaceous neoplasms. Cancer 33: 82–102
5 Troy JL, Ackerman AB (1984) Sebaceoma: A distinctive benign neoplasm of adnexal epithelium differentiating toward sebaceous cells. Am J Dermatopathol 6: 7–13

APOCRINE TUMORS

Supernumerary nipple

A supernumerary nipple appears on the anterior trunk as a soft, slightly pigmented papule along the embryonic mammary line. Histologically, components of the nipple area may be found.

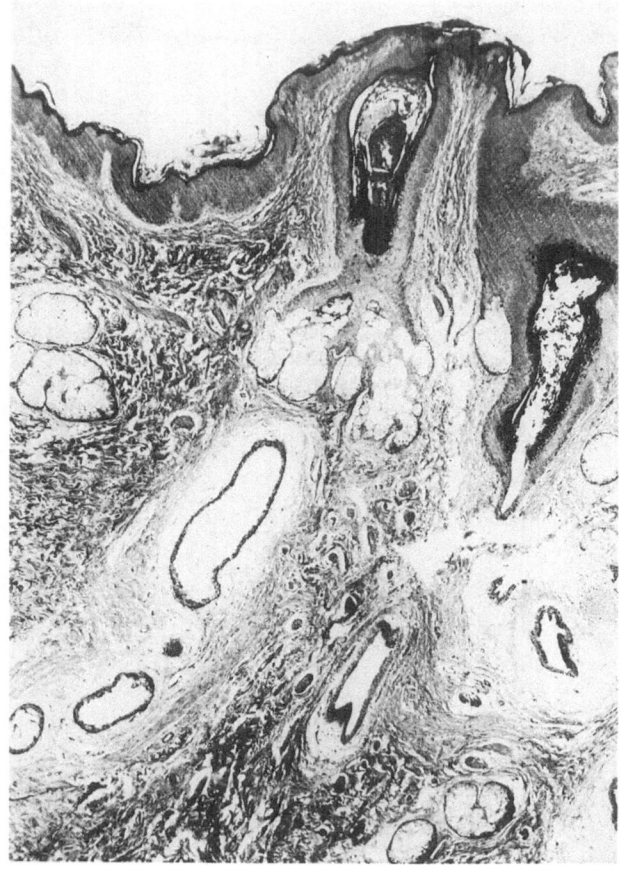

Fig. 79. Hair follicles and dilated mammary ducts are seen.
H and E, ×40

Fig. 80. Higher magnification of Fig. 79. As a characteristic feature, a large number of smooth muscles are noted. H and E, × 100

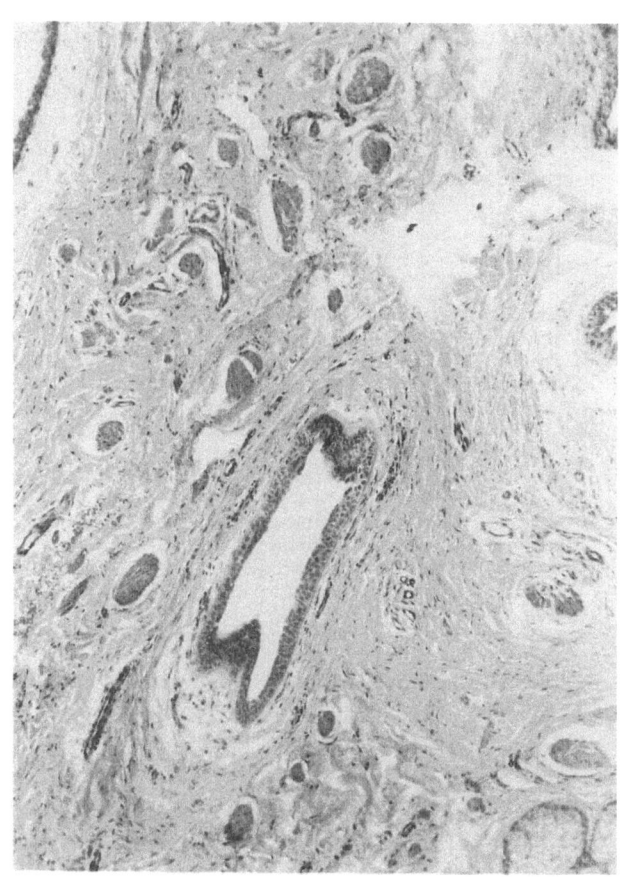

REFERENCES

1 Baruchin A. Rosenberg L (1981) A supernumerary nipple in a rare site: Report of a case. J Dermatol Surg Oncol 7: 918–919
2 Camisa C (1980) Accessory breast on the posterior thigh of a man. J Am Acad Dermatol 3: 467–469
3 Castaño M (1969) Dorsal scapular supernumerary breast in a woman: Case report. Plast Reconstr Surg 43: 536–537
4 Mehregan AH (1981) Supernumerary nipple. A histologic study. J Cutan Pathol 8: 96–104
5 Pinkus H (1964) Die makroskopische Anatomie der Haut. In: Marchionini A (ed) Handbuch der Haut- und Geschlechtskrankheiten, Ergänzungswerk, vol. 1, part 2. Springer, Berlin, pp 21–24
6 Pinkus H, Mehregan AH (1981) A guide to dermatohistopathology, 3rd edn. Appleton-Century-Crofts, New York, pp 444–445
7 Shewmake SW, Izuno GT (1977) Supernumerary areolae. Arch Dermatol 113: 823–825

Apocrine hidrocystoma, apocrine cystadenoma

Apocrine hidrocystoma is chiefly seen on the face but may occasionally be found elsewhere. As its French name *hidrocystome noir* (black hidrocystoma) suggests [7], it frequently shows pigmentation. The cause of this pigmentation is not fully understood.

REFERENCES

1 Campbell JP, Solomon AR Jr, Woo TY (1984) Apocrine cystadenoma arising in a nevus sebaceus of Jadassohn. Cutis 34: 510–512
2 Cramer HJ (1980) Das schwarze Hidrozystom (Monfort). Dermatol Monatsschr 166: 114–118
3 Hassan MO, Khan MA, Kruse TV (1979) Apocrine cystadenoma: An ultrastructural study. Arch Dermatol 115: 194–200
4 Malhotra R, Bhawan J (1985) The nature of pigment in pigmented apocrine hidrocystoma. J Cutan Pathol 12: 106–109
5 Matsumoto K, Inoue K, Fukamizu H, Moriguchi T (1983) Apocrine cystadenoma in a child. Arch Dermatol 119: 182–183
6 Mehregan AH (1964) Apocrine cystadenoma: A clinicopathologic study with special reference to the pigmented variety. Arch Dermatol 90: 274–279
7 Monfort J (1962) Les hidrocystomes noirs. Sem Hop Paris 38: 328–331
8 Murano S, Katayama J, Sakata M, Kawatsu T (1981) Apocrine cystadenoma on the back of the foot. Hifu (Osaka) 23: 226–228
9 Smith JD, Chernosky ME (1974) Apocrine hidrocystoma (Cystadenoma). Arch Dermatol 109: 700–702
10 von Seebach HB, Stumm D, Misch P, von Seebach A (1980) Hidrocystoma and adenoma of apocrine anal glands. Virchows Arch [A] 386: 231–237

Fig. 82. Higher magnification of Fig. 81. The cyst wall consists of two layers of epithelium. The inner ▷ layer shows decapitation secretion.
H and E, × 320

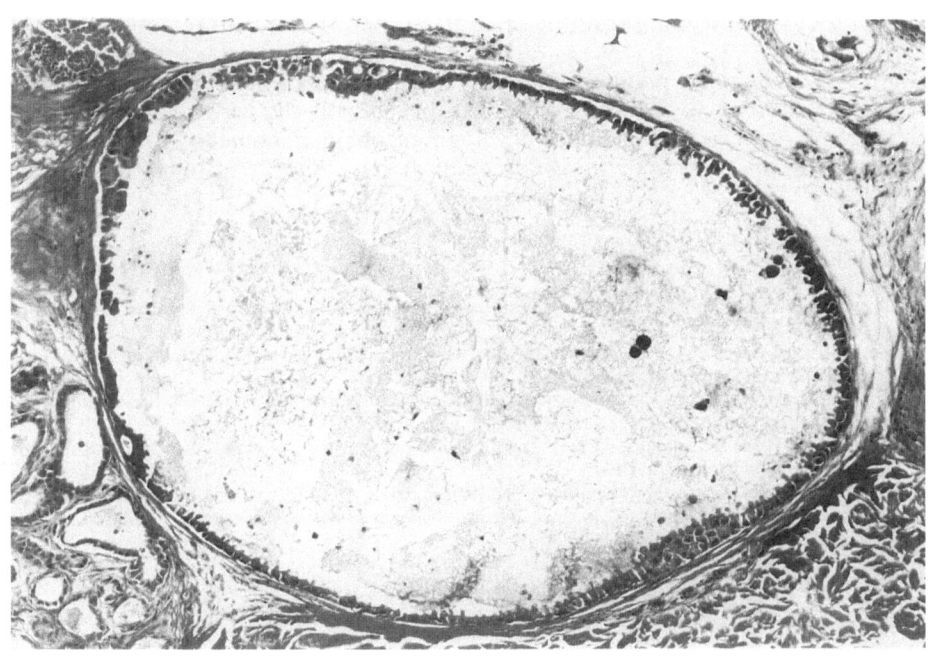

Fig. 81. This is an apocrine hidrocystoma found in syringocystadenoma papilliferum.
H and E, × 100

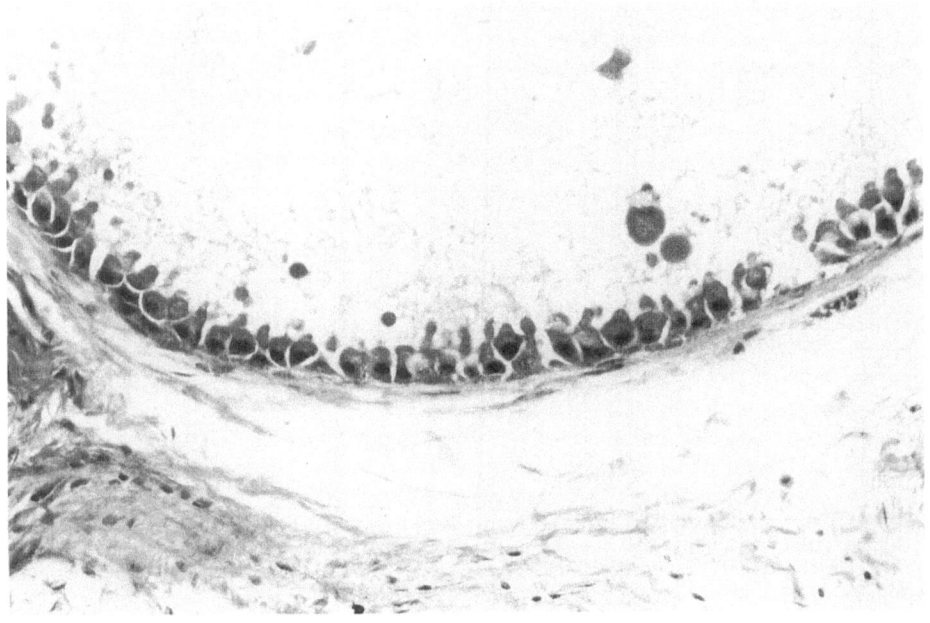

Syringocystadenoma papilliferum, syringadenoma papilliferum

Syringocystadenoma papilliferum either occurs as a primary lesion or arises at puberty within nevus sebaceus. The location is mostly the scalp or the face. There has been a rare case of this tumor developing from giant comedo [4]. The majority of these tumors show apocrine differentiation, but some are recognized as eccrine.

REFERENCES

1 Lever WF, Schaumburg-Lever G (1983) Histopathology of the skin, 6th edn. Lippincott, Philadelphia, pp 544–546
2 Mensing H, Jänner M (1981) Naevus sebaceus Jadassohn und Syringocystadenoma papilliferum: Epitheliale Hamartombildungen der Haut. Hautarzt 32: 130–135
3 Niizuma K (1976) Syringocystadenoma papilliferum: Light and electron microscopic studies. Acta Derm Venereol (Stockh) 56: 327–336
4 Niizuma K (1986) Syringocystadenoma papilliferum developed from giant comedo: A case report. Tokai J Exp Clin Med 11: 47–50
5 Pinkus H (1954) Life history of naevus syringadenomatosus papilliferus. Arch Dermatol 69: 305–322
6 Werther J (1913) Syringadenoma papilliferum (Naevus syringadenomatosus papilliferus). Arch Dermatol Syph (Berl) 116: 865–870

Fig. 84. Higher magnification of Fig. 83. The papillary structure consists of two kinds of cell—high ▷ columnar cells of the luminal side with oval nuclei and small cuboidal cells of the stromal side with round nuclei. The columnar cells show decapitation secretion (*arrow*). There are numerous plasma cells in the stroma.
H and E, × 200

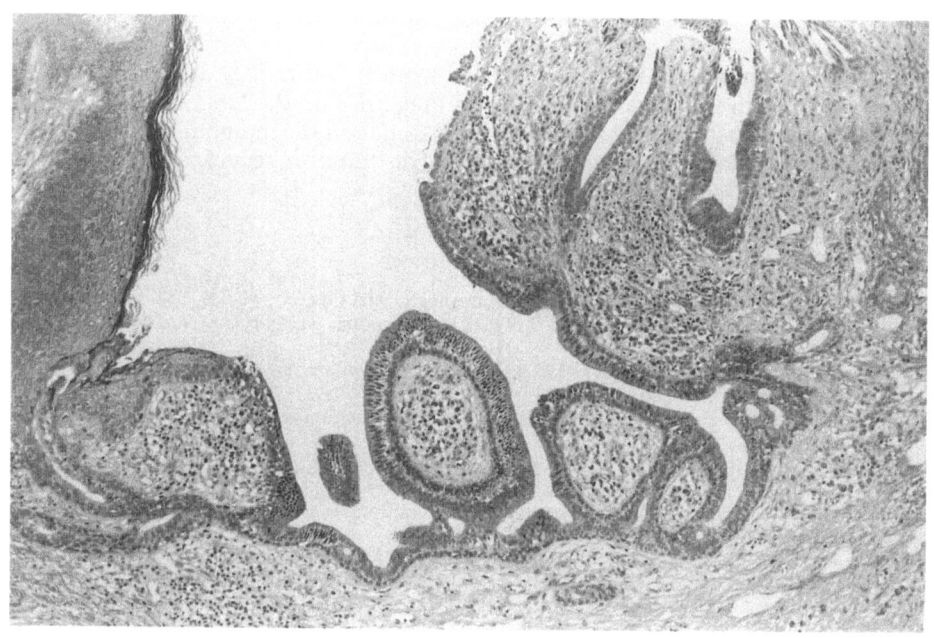

Fig. 83. This is a syringocystadenoma papilliferum found in nevus sebaceus. Papillary structures are projecting into a cystic invagination.
H and E, × 100

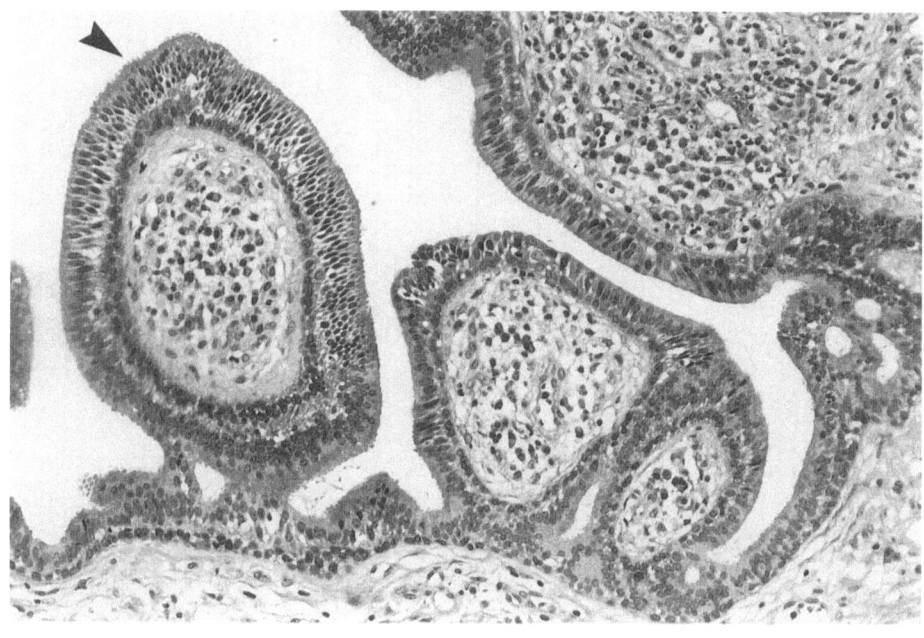

Hidradenoma papilliferum, hidradenoma of vulva

Hidradenoma papilliferum occurs only in women and mostly appears as a freely mobile nodule in the labia majora; it also may arise on the labia minora or in the perineal or perianal area. Occasionally, it is found on the mammilla, on the eyelid, and in the external auditory canal [3, 5, 6]. This tumor is regarded as apocrine.

REFERENCES

1 Ioannides G (1966) Hidradenoma papilliferum. Am J Obstet Gynecol 94: 849–853
2 Meeker JH, Neubecker RD, Helwig EB (1962) Hidradenoma papilliferum. Am J Clin Pathol 37: 182–195
3 Nissim F, Czernobilsky B, Ostfeld E (1981) Hidradenoma papilliferum of the external auditory canal. J Laryngol Otol 95: 843–848
4 Pinkus H, Mehregan AH (1981) A guide to dermatohistopathology, 3rd edn. Appleton-Century-Crofts, New York, p 447
5 Santa Cruz DJ, Prioleau PG, Smith ME (1981) Hidradenoma papilliferum of the eyelid. Arch Dermatol 117: 55–56
6 Tappeiner J, Wolff K (1968) Hidradenoma papilliferum: Eine enzymhistochemische und elektronenmikroskopische Studie. Hautarzt 19: 101–109
7 Warkel RL (1984) Selected apocrine neoplasms. J Cutan Pathol 11: 437–449
8 Woodworth H Jr, Dockerty MB, Wilson RB, Pratt JH (1971) Papillary hidradenoma of the vulva: A clinicopathologic study of 69 cases. Am J Obstet Gynecol 110: 501–508

Fig. 86. Higher magnification of Fig. 85. The stroma lacks the plasma cell infiltrate seen in syringocystadenoma papilliferum. ▷
H and E, × 200

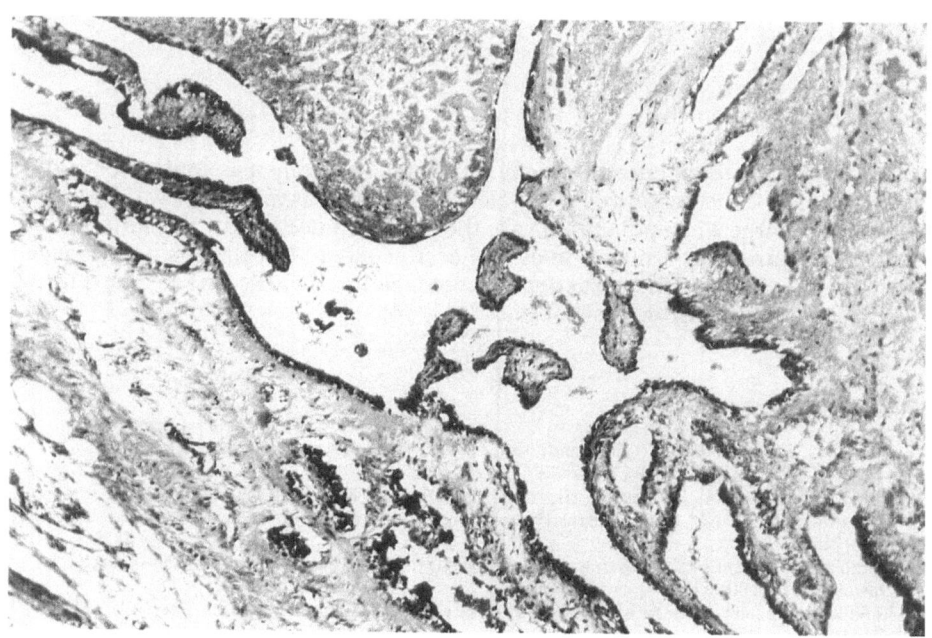

Fig. 85. Numerous thin papillary projections lined by the apocrine-type cells are protruding into the cystic cavity.
H and E, × 100

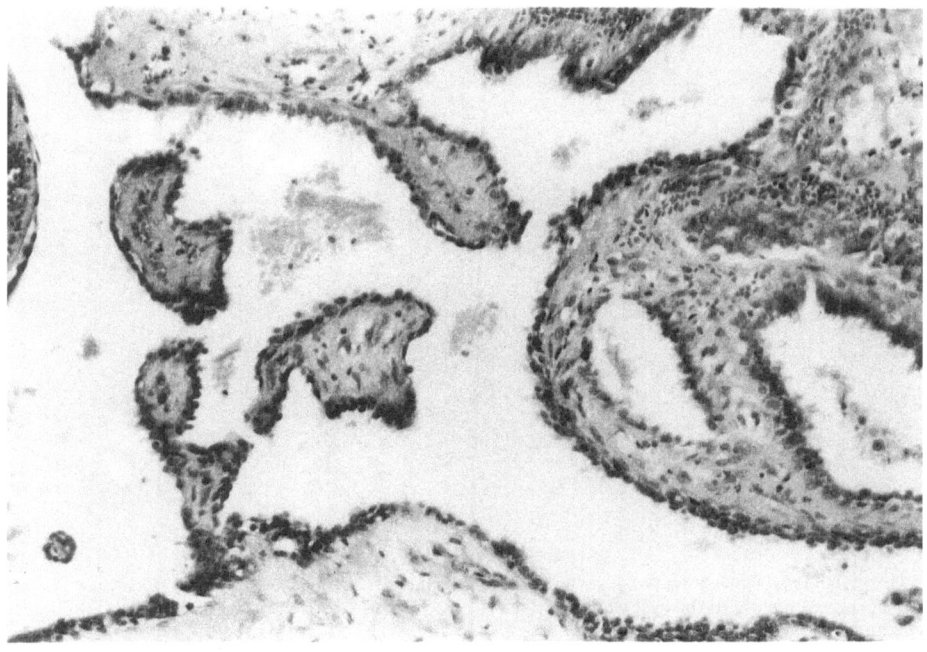

ECCRINE TUMORS

Eccrine hidrocystoma

Eccrine hidrocystoma appears chiefly on the face of women as solitary or multiple lesions. It is a translucent, cystic papule from which a drop of clear watery liquid is seen to discharge when punctured with the point of a needle. Eccrine hidrocystoma has been regarded as a retention cyst of eccrine sweat, but there is no evidence of obstruction of the eccrine sweat duct. Nevoid malformation of the eccrine duct may be involved in the histogenesis of this cyst [2, 4].

REFERENCES

1 Bures FA, Kotynek J (1982) Differentiating between apocrine and eccrine hidrocystoma. Cutis 29: 616–620
2 Ebner H, Erlach E (1975) Ekkrine Hidrozystome. Dermatol Monatsschr 161: 739–744
3 Hassan MO, Khan MA (1979) Ultrastructure of eccrine cystadenoma: A case report. Arch Dermatol 115: 1217–1221
4 Herzberg JJ (1962) Ekkrines Syringcystadenom (Hidrocystom A. R. Robinson, 1884). Arch Klin Exp Dermatol 214: 600–621
5 Maeda M, Yasuno H, Sato M (1978) A case of eccrine hidrocystoma. Acta Dermatol (Kyoto) 73: 177–180
6 Smith JD, Chernosky ME (1973) Hidrocystomas. Arch Dermatol 108: 676–679
7 Sperling LC, Sakas EL (1982) Eccrine hidrocystomas. J Am Acad Dermatol 7: 763–770

Fig. 88. The cyst wall shows two layers of flattened epithelial cells. Eccrine secretory portions and dilated ▷ ducts are seen close to the cyst wall.
H and E, × 160

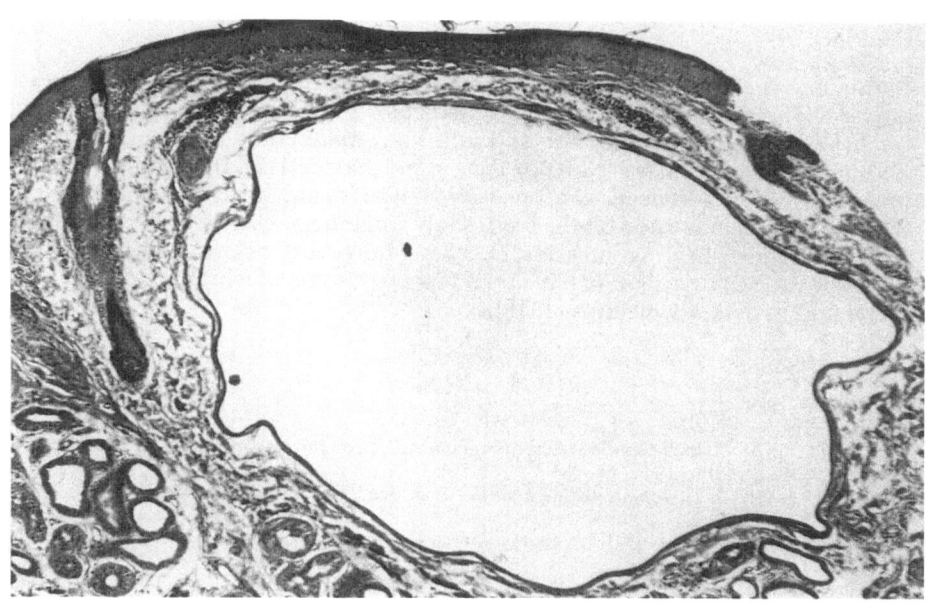

Fig. 87. Overall appearance of eccrine hidrocystoma.
H and E, ×64

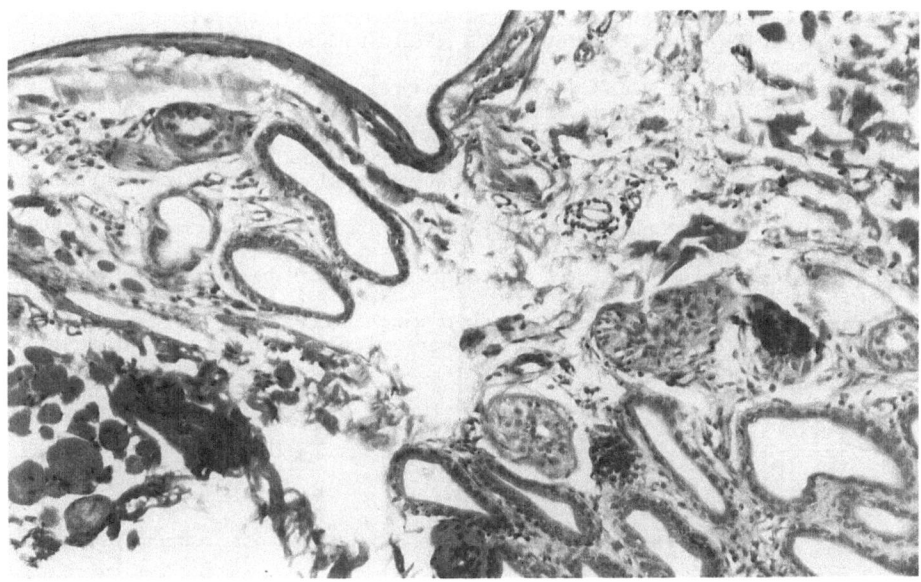

Syringoma

Syringoma is a small, skin-colored papule. As the French name *hidradénomes des paupières* (hidradenomas of the eyelids) indicates, syringomas occur predominantly on the lower eyelids, but they also appear in large numbers on the anterior chest and abdomen (*hidradénomes éruptifs* of Darier and Jacquet) [2]. In addition, they may also arise on the forehead, cheeks, neck, axillae, arms, fingers, vulva, and penis. Syringomas when located on the scalp show a plaque of cicatricial alopecia [5, 14]. The association of syringomas and Down's syndrome has been demonstrated [13]. Cases of clear cell syringoma have been reported, some of which are considered to be related to diabetes mellitus [7, 18].

REFERENCES

1 Asai Y, Ishii M, Hamada T (1982) Acral syringoma: Electron microscopic studies on its origin. Acta Derm Venereol (Stockh) 62: 64–68

2 Civatte J (1982) Histopathologie cutanée, 2nd edn. Flammarion Médecine-Science, Paris, p 275

3 Dekio S, Maehama Y (1981) Syringoma limited to genitalia of a preadolescent girl. J Dermatol (Tokyo) 8: 423–426

4 Diestelmeier MR, Rodman OG (1983) Eruptive generalized clear cell syringomas. Arch Dermatol 119: 927–929

5 Dupré A, Bonafé JL, Christol B (1981) Syringomas as a causative factor for cicatricial alopecia. Arch Dermatol 117: 315

6 Feibelman CE, Maize JC (1984) Clear-cell syringoma: A study by conventional and electron microscopy. Am J Dermatopathol 6: 139–150

7 Furue M, Hori Y, Nakabayashi Y (1984) Clear-cell syringoma: Association with diabetes mellitus. Am J Dermatopathol 6: 131–138

8 Hashimoto K, Gross BG, Lever WF (1966) Syringoma: Histochemical and electron microscopic studies. J Invest Dermatol 46: 150–166

9 Hashimoto K, Blum D, Fukaya T, Eto H (1985) Familial syringoma: Case history and application of monoclonal anti-eccrine gland antibodies. Arch Dermatol 121: 756–760

10 Hempstead RW, Hobbs ER, Howard WR (1983) Numerous syringomas of the forehead. Int J Dermatol 22: 485–486

11 Kıkuchi I, Idemori M, Okazaki M (1979) Plaque type syringoma. J Dermatol (Tokyo) 6: 329–331

12 Kitamura K, Muraki R, Tamura N (1983) Clear cell syringoma. Cutis 32: 169–172

13 Lechner W, Dötzer V (1981) Multiple Syringome bei Trisomie 21. Z Hautkr 56: 1467–1470

14 Noble JP, Lessana-Leibowitch M, Sedel D, Guillemette J, Cadot M, Hewitt J (1979) Syringome du cuir chevelu surmonté par une plaque alopécique scléro-lichénoïde. Ann Dermatol Venereol 106: 275–277

15 Tagami H, Inoue F, Yamada M, Egami K (1983) Syringoma of the forehead. Int J Dermatol 22: 113–114

16 Trozak DJ, Wood C (1984) Occult eccrine sweat duct hamartoma and cicatricial scalp alopecia. Cutis 34: 475–477

17 Weedon D (1984) Eccrine tumors: a selective review. J Cutan Pathol 11: 421–436

18 Yamasakı Y, Toda M, Kitamura K (1982) Syringomas of the clear cell type—An ultrastructural observation—J Dermatol (Tokyo) 9: 431–436

Fig. 90. The cells of the inner layer of ducts are often clear, resembling sebaceous cells. ▷ H and E, × 320

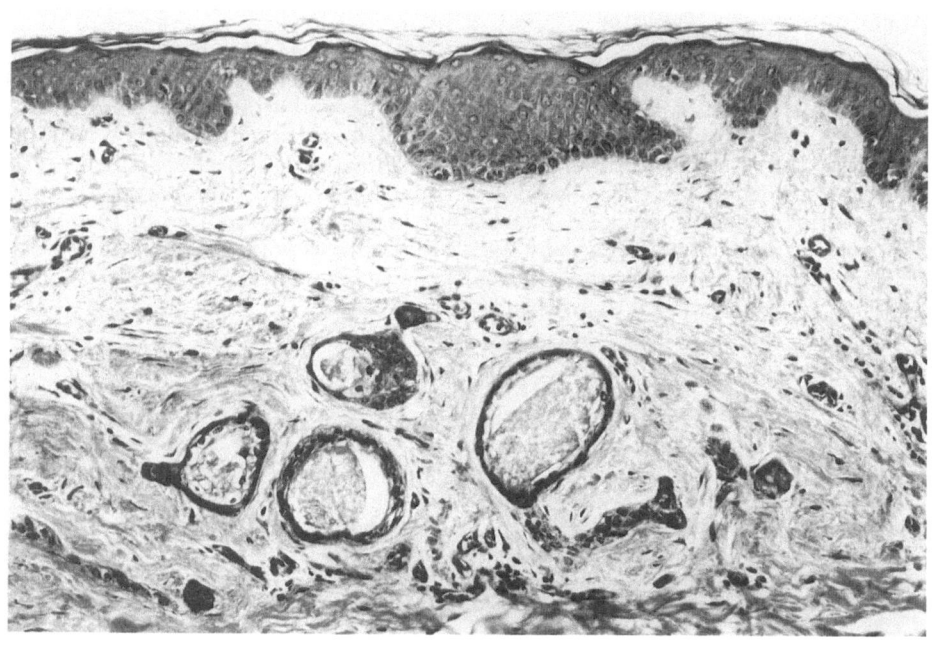

Fig. 89. Embedded in a fibrous stroma are numerous small ducts, the wall of which consists of two layers of epithelial cells. The ducts have the appearance of tadpoles.
H and E, × 160

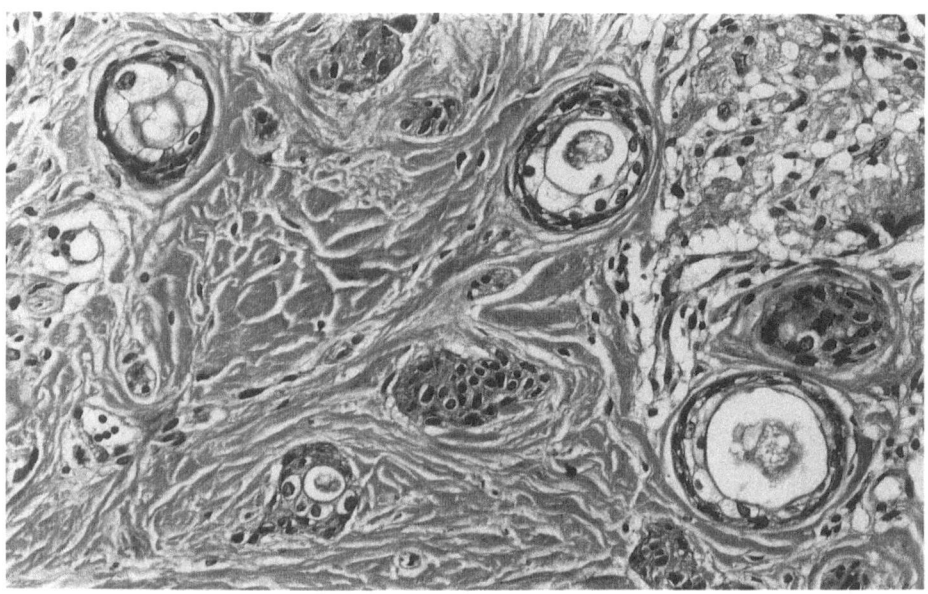

Eccrine poroma (Pinkus)

Eccrine poroma is a tumor originating from the intraepidermal eccrine sweat duct unit (acrosyringium). The tumor is a raised nodule and occurs most commonly on the soles and palms but may be seen elsewhere; it is occasionally found on the nipple [2]. Based on oncogenic differentiation, Mishima and Morioka divided eccrine poroma into three categories—eccrine poroacanthoma, eccrine poroepithelioma, and eccrine porocarcinoma [5]. "Linear eccrine poroma" reported by Ogino [6] is regarded as acrosyringeal nevus by Weedon [9]. As was pointed out by Civatte et al. [3], there are histological similarities between this type of nevus and *syringofibradénome eccrine* described by Mascaro [4].

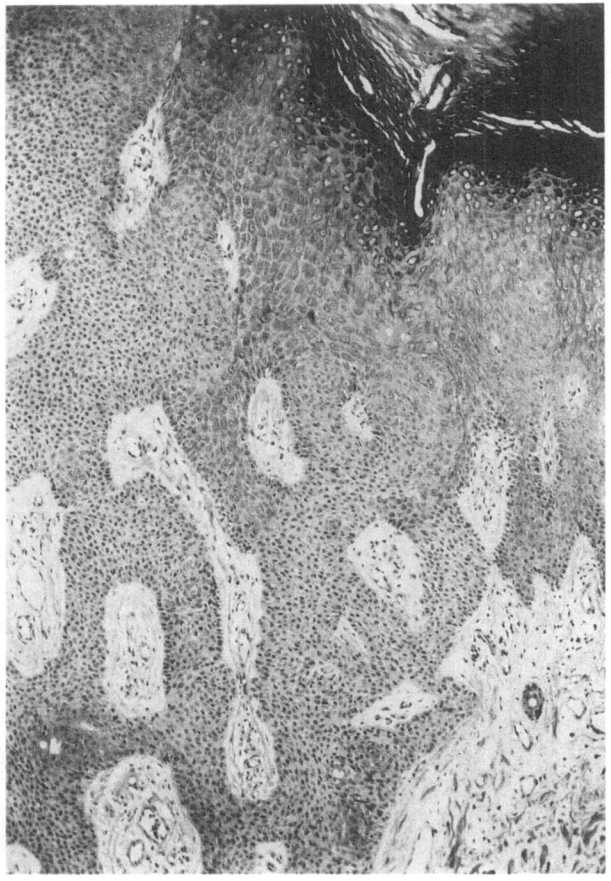

Fig. 91. Sharply demarcated from the surrounding epidermis, the tumor is seen growing. The tumor cells have a characteristic small, cuboidal appearance.
H and E, × 100

Fig. 92. A cuticle-lined lumen
is found in the tumor mass.
There is no palisade arrangement of the cells at the
periphery.
H and E, × 160

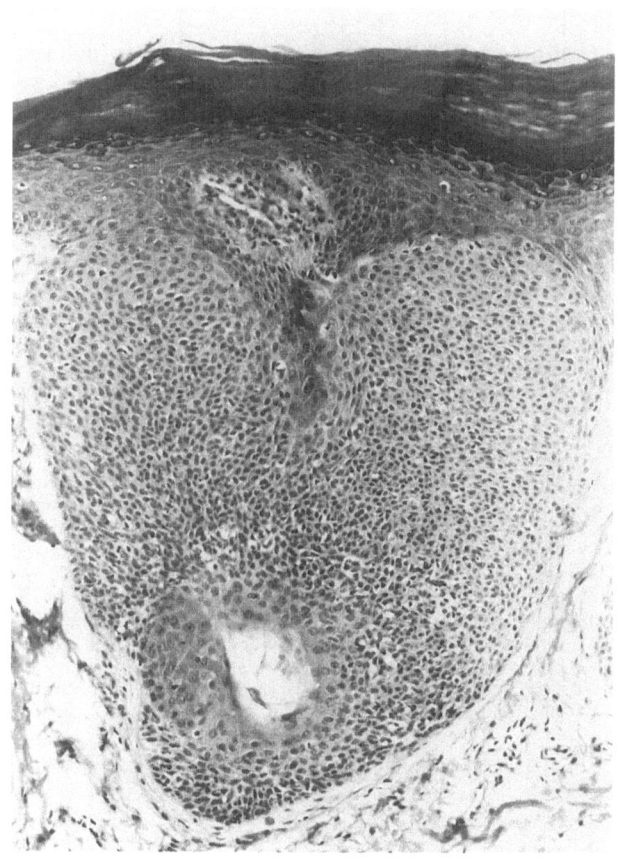

REFERENCES

1 Aoki K, Baba S, Nohara T, Suzuki H (1980) Eccrine poroma. J Dermatol (Tokyo) 7: 263–269
2 Cheon HW, Myung KB, Lee JB (1980) Eccrine poroma of the nipple. Korean J Dermatol 18: 87–91
3 Civatte J, Jeanmougin M, Barrandon Y, Jimenez de Franch A (1981) Siringofibroadenoma ecrino de Mascaró: Discusión de un caso. Med Cutan Iber Lat Am 9: 193–196
4 Mascaro JM (1963) Considérations sur les tumeurs fibro-épithéliales: Le syringofibradénome eccrine. Ann Dermatol Syph 90: 143–153
5 Mishima Y, Morioka S (1969) Oncogenic differentiation of the intraepidermal eccrine sweat duct: Eccrine poroma, poroepithelioma and porocarcinoma. Dermatologica 138: 238–250
6 Ogino A (1976) Linear eccrine poroma. Arch Dermatol 112: 841–844
7 Pinkus H, Rogin JR, Goldman P (1956) Eccrine poroma: Tumors exhibiting features of the epidermal sweat duct unit. Arch Dermatol 74: 511–521
8 Pylyser K, De Wolf-Peeters C, Marien K (1983) The histology of eccrine poromas: A study of 14 cases. Dermatologica 167: 243–249
9 Weedon D (1984) Eccrine tumors: a selective review. J Cutan Pathol 11: 421–436
10 Witkowski JA, Parish LC, Griffith CQ (1979) Solitary eccrine poroma. Int J Dermatol 18: 307–308
11 Yasuda T, Kawada A, Yoshida K (1964) Eccrine poroma: A Japanese case showing melanin granules and melanocytes in the tumor. Arch Dermatol 90: 428–431

Hidroacanthoma simplex (Smith and Coburn)

Smith and Coburn reassessed the tumors which in the past had been diagnosed as intraepidermal epithelioma of Borst-Jadassohn, and they confirmed the eccrine nature of the intraepidermal nest formation in some tumors of this type. Thus, Smith and Coburn introduced the term "hidroacanthoma simplex" [10].

REFERENCES

1 Cook MG, Ridgway HA (1979) The intra-epidermal epithelioma of Jadassohn: a distinct entity. Br J Dermatol 101: 659–667
2 Holubar K, Wolff K (1969) Intra-epidermal eccrine poroma: A histochemical and enzyme-histo-chemical study. Cancer 23: 626–635
3 Ishikawa K (1971) Malignant hidroacanthoma simplex. Arch Dermatol 104: 529–532
4 Kennedy C, Bhogal B, Moss R, Sanderson KV (1979) Pigmented intraepidermal eccrine poroma. Br J Dermatol 101 (Suppl 17): 76–78
5 Kitamura K, Kinehara M, Tamura N, Nakamura K (1983) Hidroacanthoma simplex with invasive growth. Cutis 32: 83–88
6 Mehregan AH, Pinkus H (1964) Intraepidermal epithelioma: A critical study. Cancer 17: 609–636
7 Mehregan AH, Levson DN (1969) Hidroacanthoma simplex: A report of two cases. Arch Dermatol 100: 303–305
8 Oka K, Morohashi M, Nitto H (1975) Hidroacanthoma simplex: An ultrastructural study and comparison with eccrine poroma. J Dermatol (Tokyo) 2: 69–78
9 Rahbari H (1983) Hidroacanthoma simplex—a review of 15 cases. Br J Dermatol 109: 219–225
10 Smith JLS, Coburn JG (1956) Hidroacanthoma simplex: An assessment of a selected group of intraepidermal basal cell epitheliomata and of their malignant homologues. Br J Dermatol 68: 400–418
11 Warner TFCS, Goell WS, Cripps DJJ (1982) Hidroacanthoma simplex: an ultrastructural study. J Cutan Pathol 9: 189–195

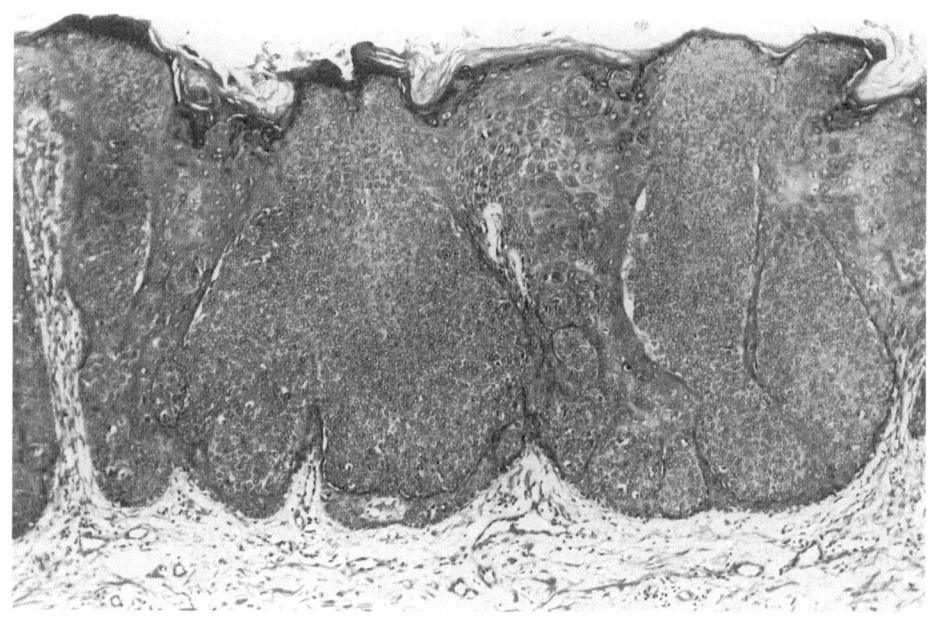

Fig. 93. Nests consisting of eccrine poromalike cells are seen confined within the epidermis. H and E, × 100

Dermal duct tumor (Winkelmann and McLeod)

Dermal duct tumor is a papule or nodule without characteristic clinical features that occurs mostly in women. Histologically, solid tumor masses of various size are seen almost entirely in the dermis; they consist of the same cells as those in eccrine poroma.

REFERENCES

1 Apisarnthanarax P, Mullins JF (1975) Dermal duct tumor. Arch Dermatol 111: 1171–1173
2 Cramer HJ (1972) Ekkrines Ductom. Zentralbl Allg Pathol 115: 113–118
3 Degos R, Civatte J, Belaïch S, Tsoïtis G (1969) "Dermal duct tumor" de Winkelmann et McLeod (Un cas). Bull Soc Fr Dermatol Syph 76: 59–62
4 Enjoji M, Tashiro M (1968) Dermal duct tumor: A variant of eccrine poroma. Acta Med Univ Kagoshima 10: 85–90
5 Faure M, Colomb D (1979) Dermal duct tumor. J Cutan Pathol 6: 317–322
6 Hu CH, Marques AS, Winkelmann RK (1978) Dermal duct tumor: A histochemical and electron microscopic study. Arch Dermatol 114: 1659–1664
7 Ishikawa K (1976) Dermal duct tumour. Australas J Dermatol 17: 30–32
8 Mishima Y (1969) Epitheliomatous differentiation of the intraepidermal eccrine sweat duct: Eccrine poroepithelioma revealed by electron microscopy. J Invest Dermatol 52: 233–246
9 Nagao S, Sonoda K (1974) Light and electron microscopic observations of eccrine poroepithelioma (Dermal duct tumor). Med J Aomori 19: 399–409
10 Winkelmann RK, McLeod WA (1966) The dermal duct tumor. Arch Dermatol 94: 50–55

Fig. 95. Higher magnification of Fig. 94. A small ductal lumen is seen in the tumor mass. There is no ▷ peripheral palisading of the tumor cells.
H and E, × 200

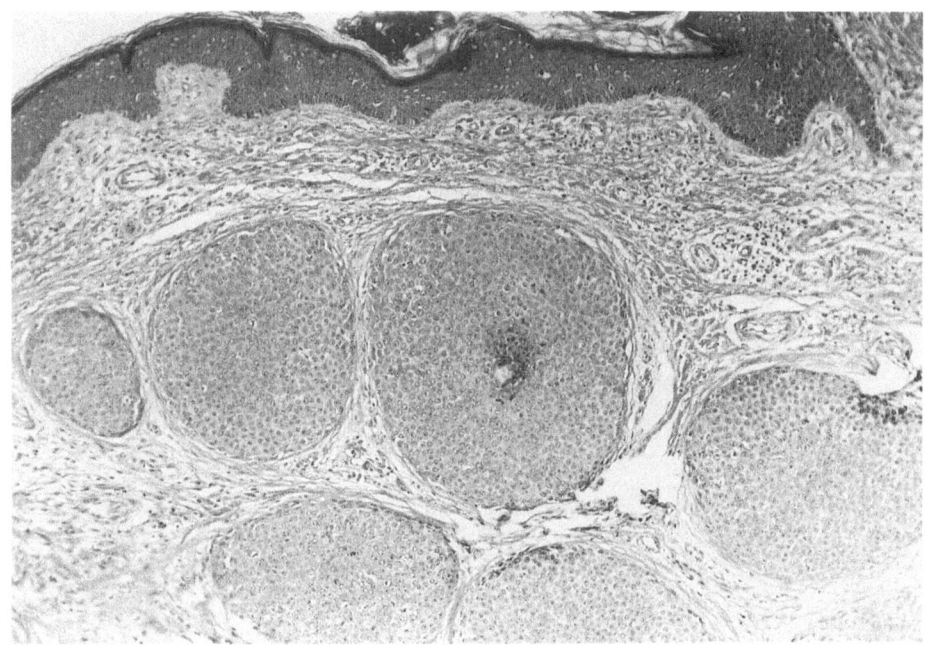

Fig. 94. The upper part of dermal duct tumor.
H and E, × 100

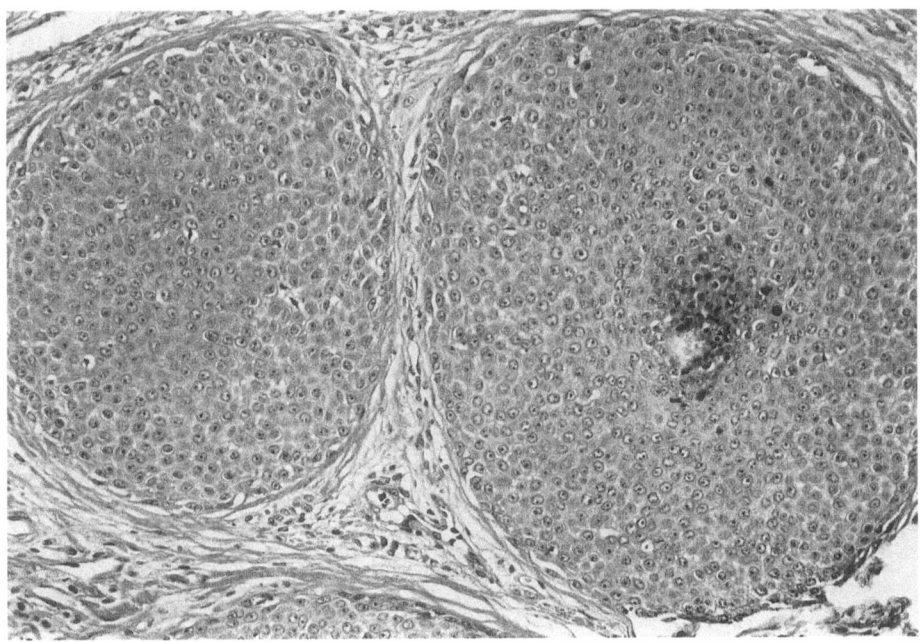

Eccrine spiradenoma

Eccrine spiradenoma is a nodule in the dermis. There is no common site. The tumor is often painful.

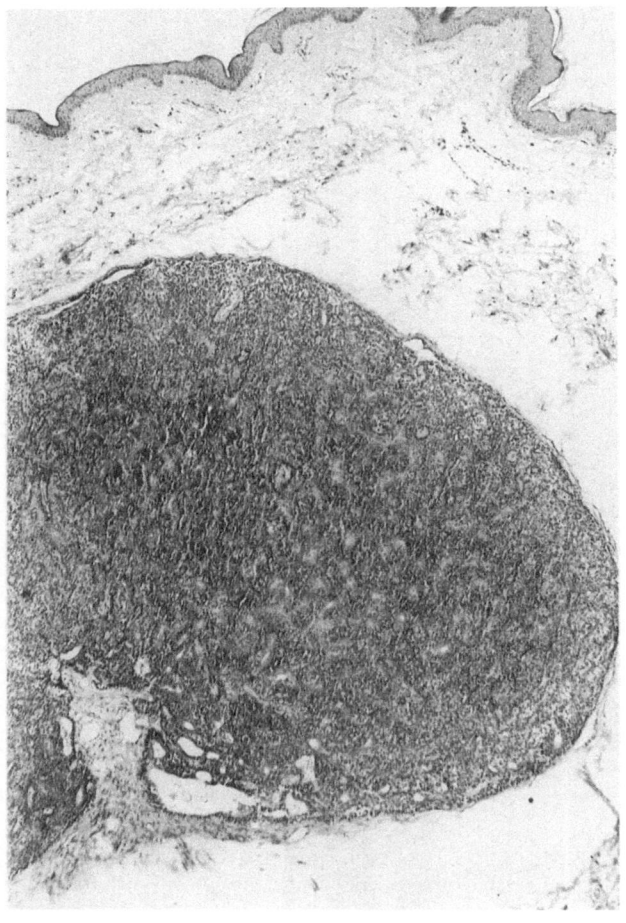

Fig 96. A large tumor mass is seen, which is deeply basophilic and has small lumina. H and E, × 64

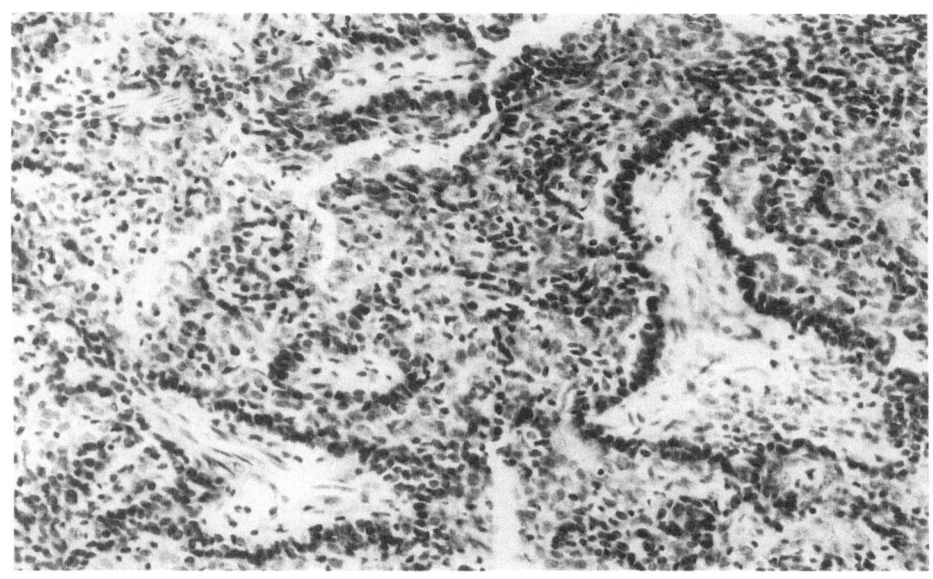

Fig. 97. The tumor consists of intertwining cords of epithelial cells, enclosing the stroma. Two kinds of epithelial cell are evident—cells with small, dark nuclei, lying at the periphery of the cords and cells with large, pale nuclei, lying in the center of the cords or around small lumina. In addition, a rosettelike arrangement of the latter cells is regarded as a characteristic of this tumor [1, 3, 5].
H and E, × 320

REFERENCES

1 Burgdorf WHC, Nasemann Th, Jänner M, Schütte B (1984) Dermatopathology. Springer, New York, p 158
2 Eich N, Lechner W (1985) Das ekkrine Spiradenom. Hautarzt 36: 240–241
3 Hornstein OP, Weidner F (1979) Tumoren der Haut. In: Doerr W, Seifert G, Uehlinger E (eds) Spezielle pathologische Anatomie: Ein Lehr-und Nachschlagewerk, 2nd edn., vol. 7, part 2. Springer, Berlin, pp 170–172
4 Kersting DW, Helwig EB (1956) Eccrine spiradenoma. Arch Dermatol 73: 199–227
5 Lever WF, Schaumburg-Lever G (1983) Histopathology of the skin, 6th edn. Lippincott, Philadelphia, pp 555–557
6 Mambo NC (1983) Eccrine spiradenoma: clinical and pathologic study of 49 tumors. J Cutan Pathol 10: 312–320

Clear cell hidradenoma

REFERENCES

1 Beck HG, Lechner W (1985) Klarzellenhidradenom. Aktuel Dermatol 11: 171–172
2 Hashimoto K, DiBella RJ, Lever WF (1967) Clear cell hidradenoma: Histological, histochemical, and electron microscopic studies. Arch Dermatol 96: 18–38
3 Helwig EB (1984) Eccrine acrospiroma. J Cutan Pathol 11: 415–420
4 Hernández-Pérez E, Cestoni-Parducci R (1985) Nodular hidradenoma and hidradenocarcinoma: A 10-year review. J Am Acad Dermatol 12: 15–20
5 Keasbey LE, Hadley GG (1954) Clear-cell hidradenoma: Report of three cases with widespread metastases. Cancer 7: 934–952
6 Lever WF, Schaumburg-Lever G (1983) Histopathology of the skin, 6th edn. Lippincott, Philadelphia, pp 557–560
7 Tezuka T, Kikuchi A, Seiji M (1968) Clear cell hidradenoma. Jpn J Dermatol Ser B 78: 287–302
8 Schütte B, Jänner M (1979) Klarzellenhidradenom ungewöhnlicher Lokalisation. Hautarzt 30: 264–266

Fig. 99. Higher magnification. There is no palisading of cells at the periphery of the tumor lobules. ▷
H and E, × 200

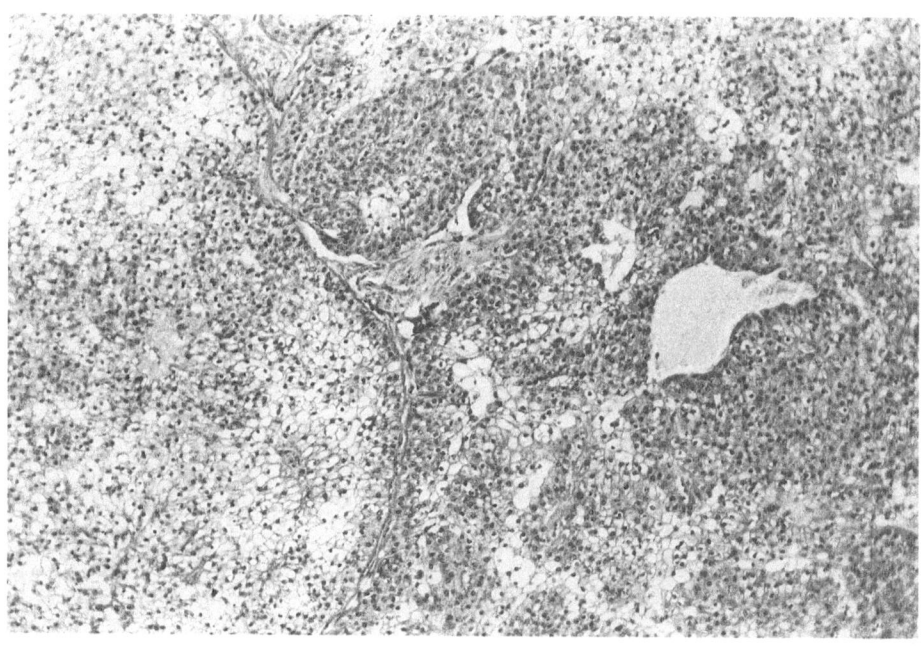

Fig. 98. In this type of nodular hidradenoma, numerous clear cells are seen in lobulated tumor masses, which contain cystic spaces.
H and E, × 100

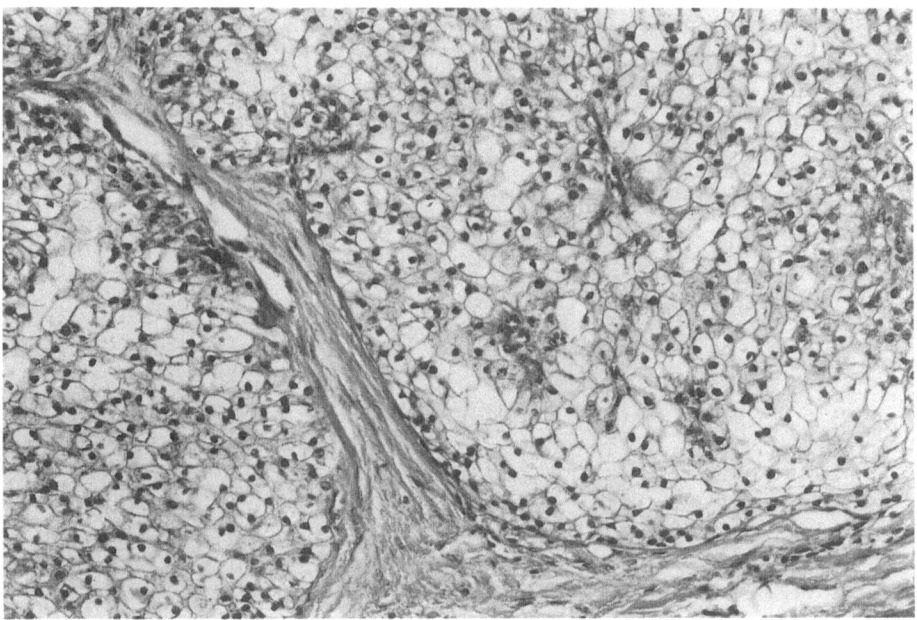

Solid-cystic hidradenoma (Winkelmann and Wolff)

Solid-cystic hidradenoma is a type of nodular hidradenoma. It may arise in any part of the body.

REFERENCES

1 Brownstein MH, Shapiro L (1975) The sweat gland adenomas. Int J Dermatol 14: 397–411
2 Stanley RJ, Sanchez NP, Massa MC, Cooper AJ, Crotty CP, Winkelmann RK (1982) Epidermoid hidradenoma. A clinicopathologic study. J Cutan Pathol 9: 293–302
3 Winkelmann RK, Wolff K (1968) Solid-cystic hidradenoma of the skin: Clinical and histopathologic study. Arch Dermatol 97: 651–661
4 Wolff K, Winkelmann RK, Decker RH (1968) Solid-cystic hidradenoma: An enzyme histochemical, biochemical, and electron microscopic study. Acta Dermatol (Kyoto) 63: 309–322

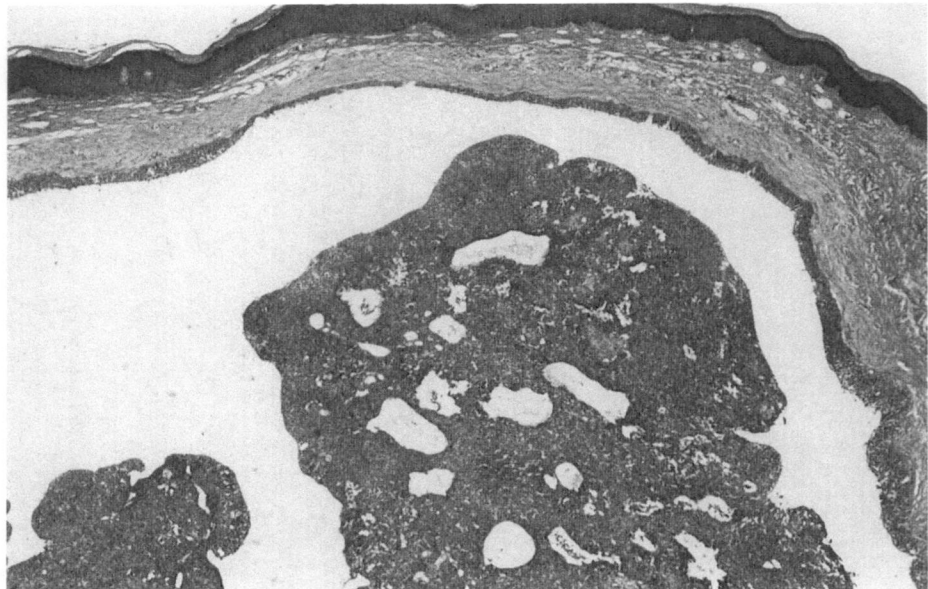

Fig. 100. A solid tumor mass is seen and appears to be growing into a large cystic cavity. H and E, × 32

Fig. 101. Most of the tumor
cells are epidermoid in
appearance.
H and E, × 320

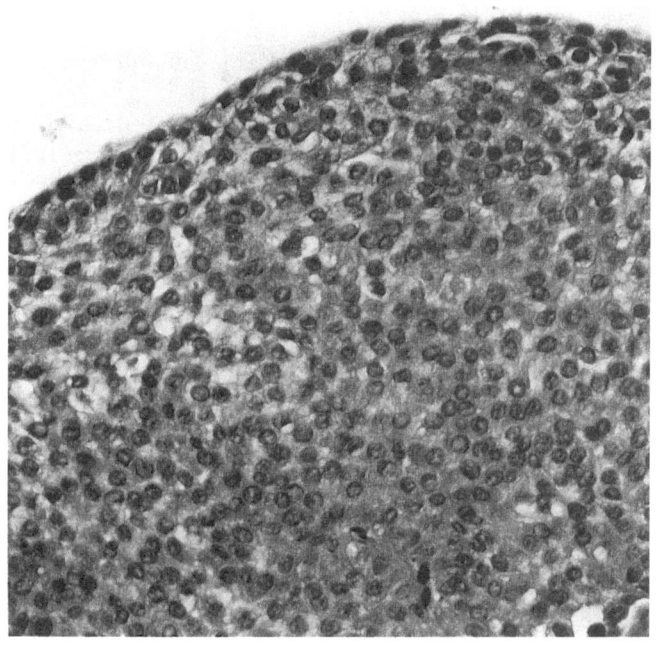

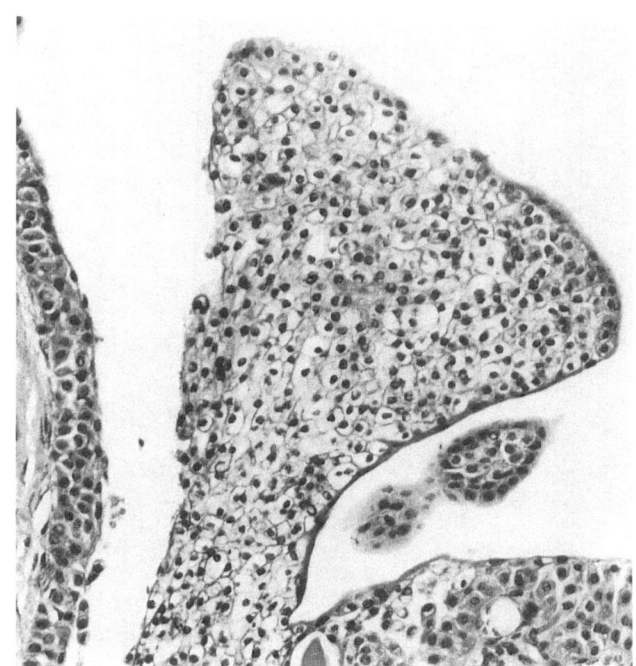

Fig. 102. A group of clear
cells are evident.
H and E, × 200

Chondroid syringoma (Hirsch and Helwig), mixed tumor of the skin

Chondroid syringoma is an intradermal nodule found mostly on the head and neck, but it does occur elsewhere on the body [1, 2, 5, 9]. Because the overlying skin appears normal, it is not infrequently misdiagnosed as a cyst. Histologically, however, it generally has the ductal structures suggestive of eccrine differentiation; cases showing a ductal lumina of the apocrine type have also been recognized [1, 10].

REFERENCES

1 Haensch R (1983) Apokriner Mischtumor. Z Hautkr 58: 575–579
2 Hirsch P, Helwig EB (1961) Chondroid syringoma: Mixed tumor of skin, salivary gland type. Arch Dermatol 84: 835–847
3 Jaimovich L, Arcuri S, Tognaccioli O, Zeitlin E, Woscoff A (1984) Chondroid syringoma. J Dermatol (Tokyo) 11: 570–576
4 Maekawa Y, Nogita T, Arao T (1985) Two cases of so-called mixed tumor of the skin—Distribution of fibronectin and laminin in the stroma—Nishinihon J Dermatol 47: 220–223
5 Mambo NC (1984) Hyaline cells in a benign chondroid syringoma: Report of a case and findings by conventional and electron microscopy. Am J Dermatopathol 6: 265–272

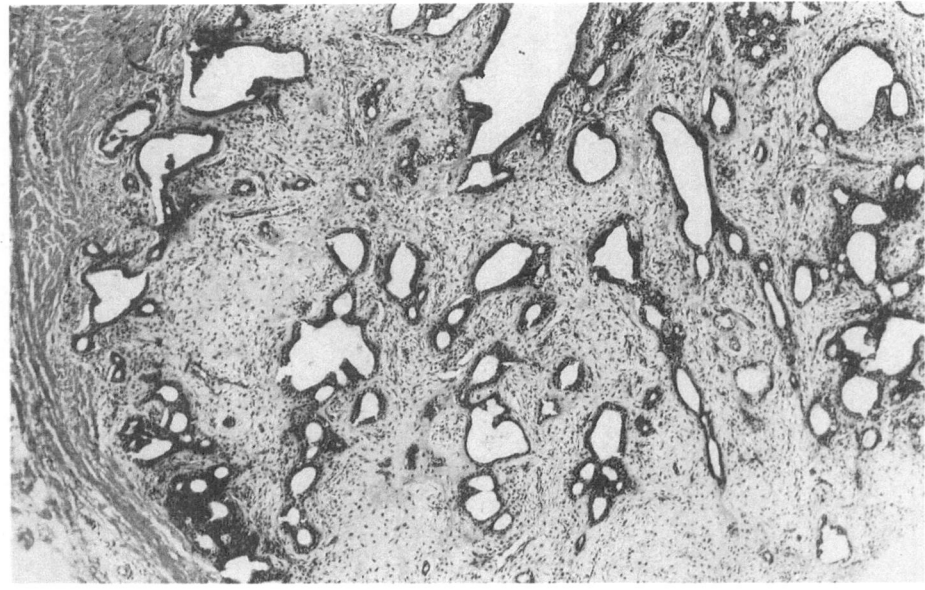

Fig. 103. Numerous branching, tubular lumina are embedded in a strongly mucoid stroma. H and E, × 64

Fig. 104. Higher magnification of Fig. 103. The tubular lumina are lined by two layers of epithelial cells. H and E, × 160

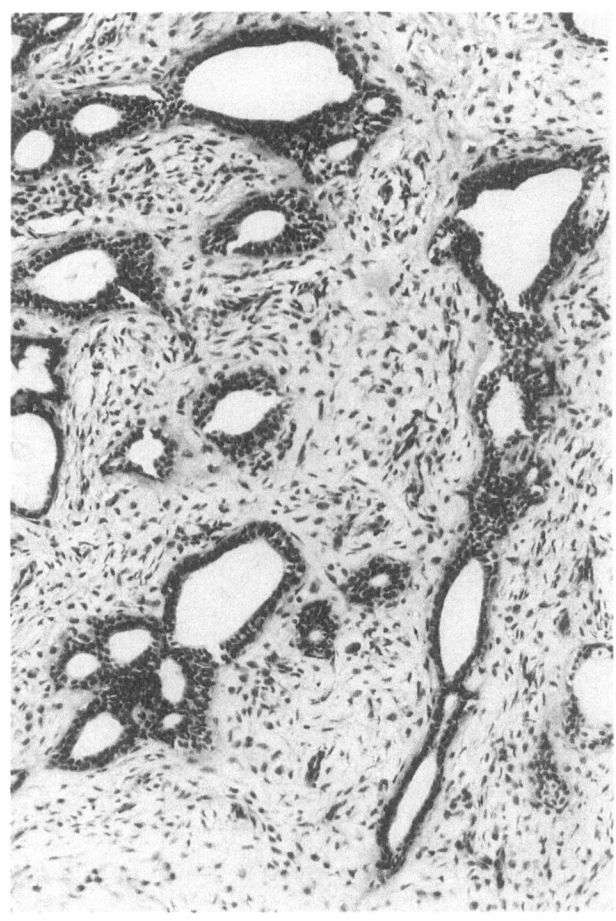

6 Masuda T, Ikeda S (1965) So-called mixed tumors of the skin of salivary gland type. Jpn J Dermatol Ser B 75: 37–43
7 Mills SE (1984) Mixed tumor of the skin: a model of divergent differentiation. J Cutan Pathol 11: 382–386
8 Rapini RP, Kennedy LJ, Golitz LE (1984) Hair matrix differentiation in chondroid syringoma. J Cutan Pathol 11: 318–321
9 Solanki RL, Ramdeo IN, Goyal AK (1979) Chondroid syringoma. (Mixed tumour of skin—Salivary gland type—Report of four cases). Indian J Dermatol Venereol Lepr 45: 59–62
10 Welke S, Goos M (1982) Das chondroide Syringom. Hautarzt 33: 15–17

BASAL CELL EPITHELIOMA

Solid basal cell epithelioma

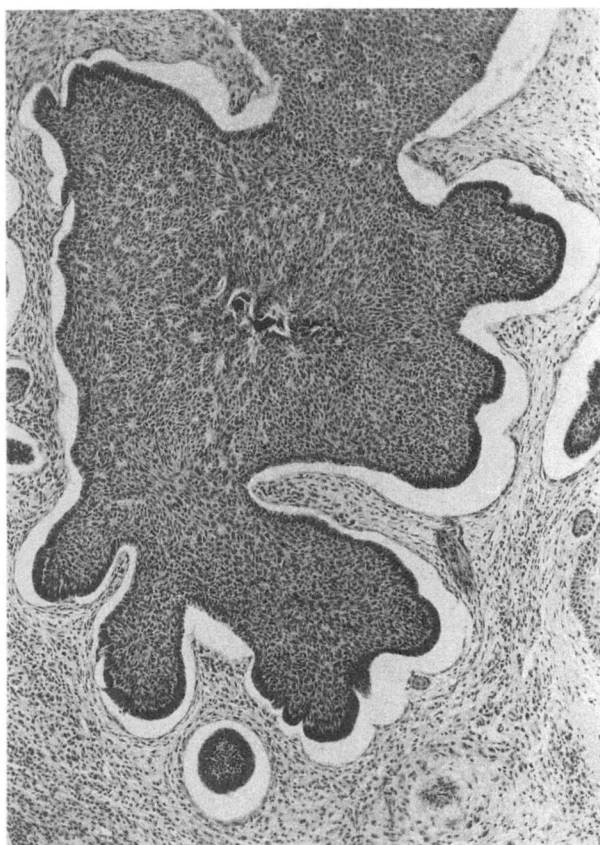

Fig. 105. There is a large, solid, irregularly outlined mass of basalioma cells. The peripheral cell layer shows a palisade arrangement. Retraction of the stroma from the tumor mass is seen. H and E, × 100

Keratotic basal cell epithelioma

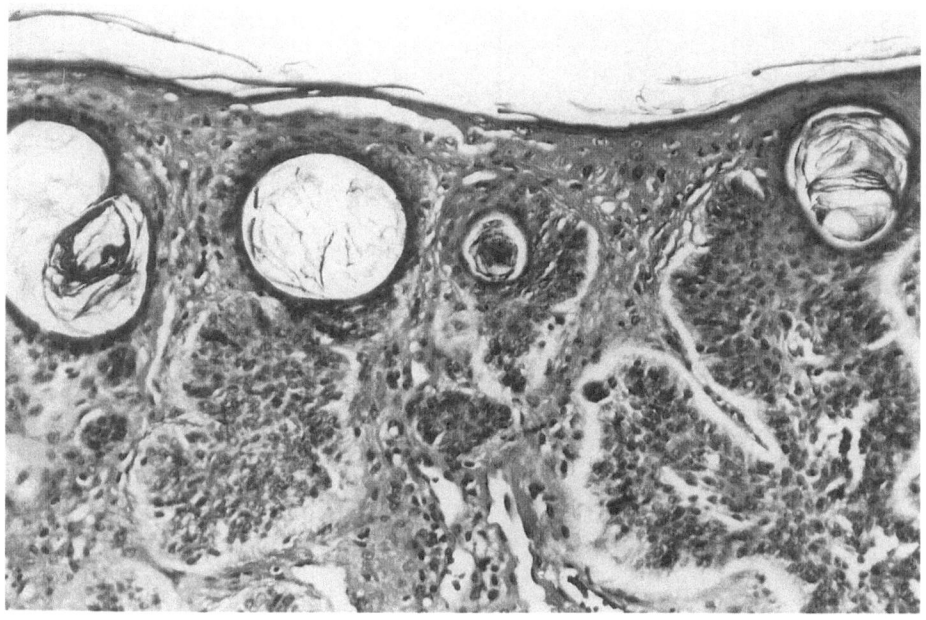

Fig. 106. Horn cysts are seen in the tumor masses. They show keratinization without the formation of the granular cells.
H and E, × 200

Adenoid basal cell epithelioma

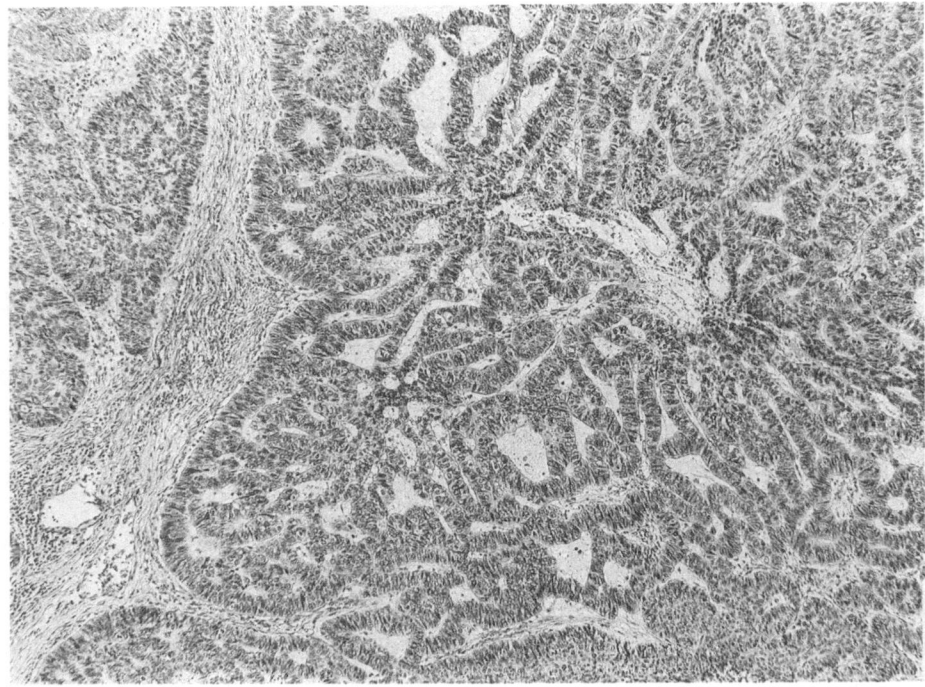

Fig. 107. A lacelike arrangement of tumor cells is characteristic of this type of basal cell epithelioma. H and E, × 80

Cystic (or pseudocystic) basal cell epithelioma

According to Kint, this cystic change of basal cell epithelioma is formed in three ways: (1) by extension of stellar atrophy, (2) massive necrosis of tumor cells, or (3) destructed stroma enclosed completely within the tumor mass [1–3].

REFERENCES

1 Kint A (1970) Histogenetic study of the basal cell epithelioma. Curr Probl Dermatol 3: 82–123
2 Kint A (1974) Die Histogenese des Basalioms. Hautarzt 25: 521–527
3 Kint A (1976) Pathology of basal cell epithelioma. In: Andrade R, Gumport SL, Popkin GL, Rees TD (eds) Cancer of the skin: Biology-diagnosis-management. Saunders, Philadelphia, pp 845–882

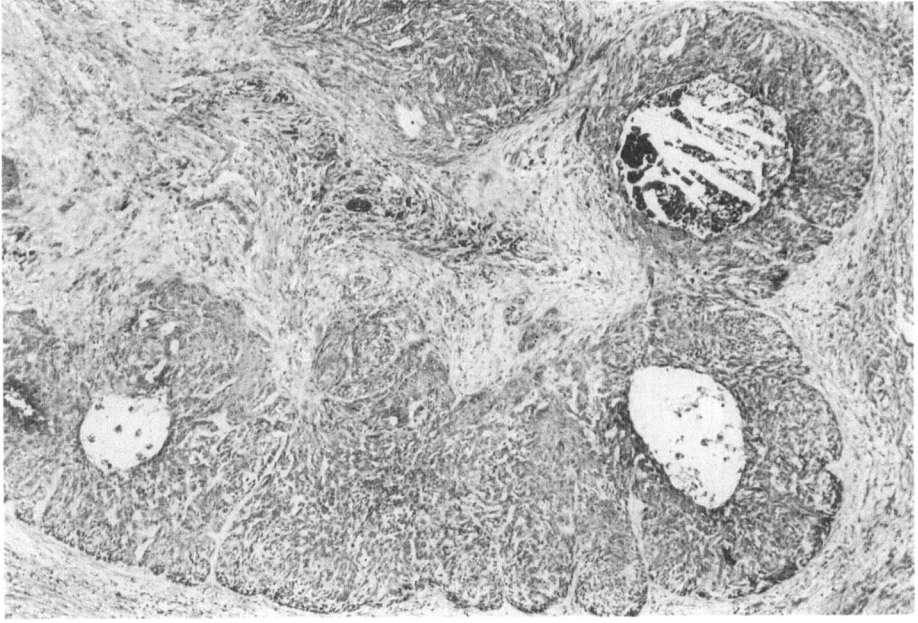

Fig. 108. In the tumor masses, there are cystic cavities showing no keratinization. H and E, × 64

Sclerosing basal cell epithelioma

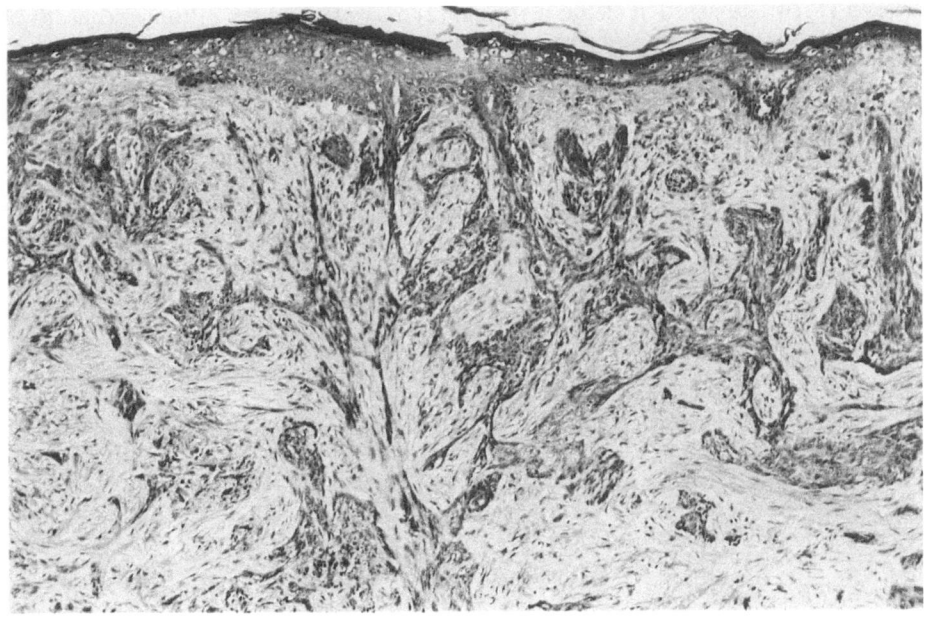

Fig. 109. Narrow, branching strands of basalioma cells are embedded in an ample, fibrous stroma. H and E, × 100

REFERENCES

1 Pinkus H, Mehregan AH (1981) A guide to dermatohistopathology, 3rd edn. Appleton-Century-Crofts, New York, p 461
2 Sloane JP (1977) The value of typing basal cell carcinomas in predicting recurrence after surgical excision. Br J Dermatol 96: 127–132

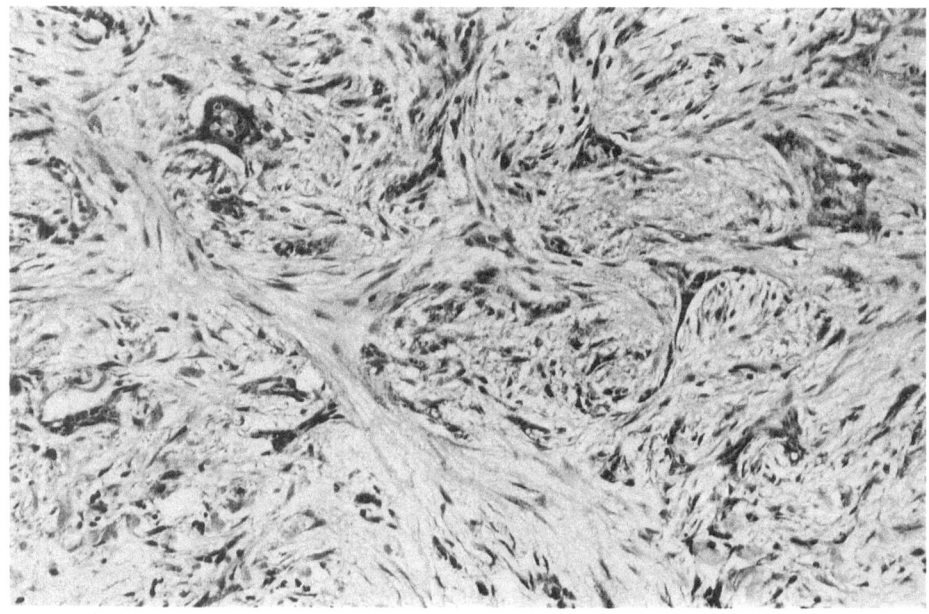

Fig. 110. Small, thin, branching cords of the tumor cells are embedded in an overabundant fibrous stroma. H and E, × 200

Stellar atrophy or adamantinoid pattern of basal cell epithelioma

Though the intercellular bridges are best seen electron microscopically in basal cell epithelioma [9], they are occasionally detectable with light microscopy [10]. If a mucoid substance accumulates in the intercellular spaces, the closely packed basalioma cells become widely separated and interconnected by elongated cytoplasmic processes and stretched intercellular bridges, giving the tumor cells a starlike appearance. The palisade arrangement of the peripheral cells is, however, preserved. This histological change is called stellar atrophy or adamantinoid pattern of basal cell epithelioma.

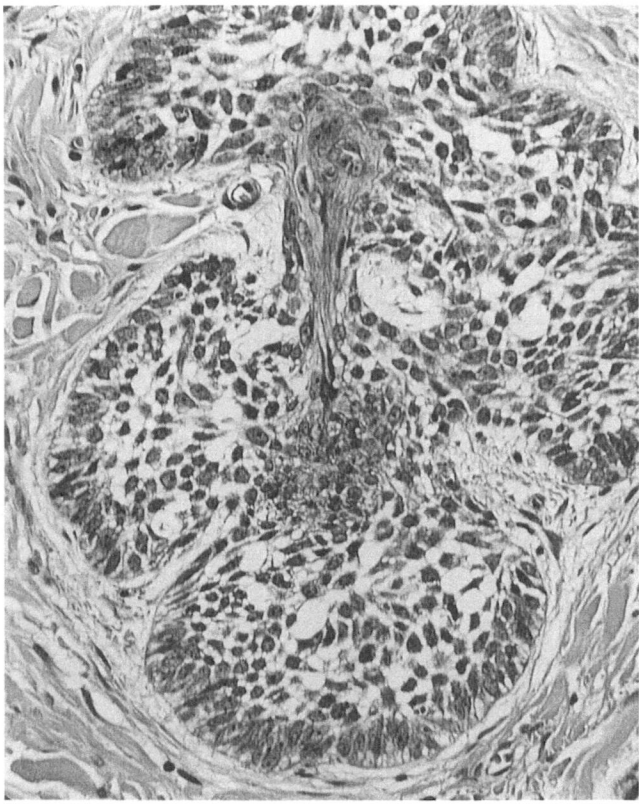

Fig. 111. The intercellular spaces are wide but the basalioma cells are interconnected and have a starlike appearance. Peripheral palisading of the cells is evident. H and E, × 320

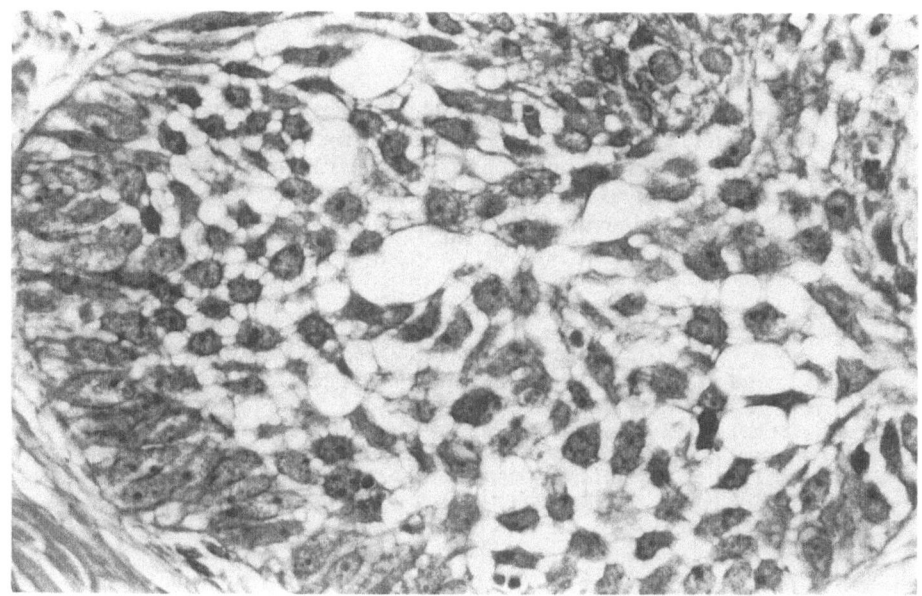

Fig. 112. High magnification of Fig. 111. The tumor cells are seen interconnected by elongated cytoplasmic processes and intercellular bridges.
H and E, × 800

REFERENCES

1 Civatte J (1982) Histopathologie cutanée, 2nd edn Flammarion Médecine-Science, Paris, p 324

2 Hornstein OP, Weidner F (1979) Tumoren der Haut. In: Doerr W. Seifert G, Uehlinger E (eds) Spezielle pathologische Anatomie: Ein Lehr-und Nachschlagewerk, 2nd edn, vol. 7, part 2. Springer, Berlin, pp 193–196

3 Kint A (1970) Histogenetic study of the basal cell epithelioma. Curr Probl Dermatol 3: 82–123

4 Kint A (1974) Die Histogenese des Basalioms. Hautarzt 25: 521–527

5 Kint A (1976) Pathology of basal cell epithelioma. In: Andrade R, Gumport SL, Popkin GL, Rees TD (eds) Cancer of the skin: Biology-diagnosis-management. Saunders, Philadelphia, pp 845–882

6 Lerchin E, Rahbari H (1975) Adamantinoid basal cell epithelioma: A histological variant. Arch Dermatol 111: 586–588

7 Lever WF, Schaumburg-Lever G (1983) Histopathology of the skin, 6th edn. Lippincott, Philadelphia, p 568

8 Pinkus H, Mehregan AH (1981) A guide to dermatohistopathology, 3rd edn. Appleton-Century-Crofts, New York, pp 458–459

9 Reidbord HE, Wechsler HL, Fisher ER (1971) Untrastructural study of basal cell carcinoma and its variants with comments on histogenesis. Arch Dermatol 104: 132–140

10 Schwartz RA, Hansen RC, Maize JC (1980) The blue-gray cystic basal cell epithelioma. J Am Acad Dermatol 2: 155–160

Superficial basal cell epithelioma, épithéliome pagétoïde, Rumpfhautepitheliom

This type of basal cell epithelioma often has a peculiar clinical appearance. As described by Darier, the lesion is a well-circumscribed round plaque and is bordered by a fine, threadlike elevation or by papules (*perles*) arranged like a string of beads [1]. The location is mostly the trunk. The histological growth mode of this tumor is closely related to premalignant fibroepithelial tumor [4].

REFERENCES

1 Darier J (1928) Précis de dermatologie, 4th edn. Masson, Paris, pp 978–983
2 Madsen A (1955) The histogenesis of superficial basal-cell epitheliomas: Unicentric or multicentric origin. Arch Dermatol 72: 29–30
3 Madsen A (1965) Studies on basal-cell epithelioma of the skin. The architecture, manner of growth, and histogenesis of the tumours. Whole tumours examined in serial sections cut parallel to the skin surface. Acta Pathol Microbiol Scand (Suppl) 177: 1–63
4 Pinkus H (1965) Epithelial and fibroepithelial tumors. Arch Dermatol 91: 24–37

Fig. 113. Embedded in an ample, fine-fibrous, myxomatous stroma, numerous irregular masses of ▷ basalioma cells are seen growing down from the undersurface of the epidermis; the cells áre superficially localized in the pars reticularis of the dermis. Since the tumor cells are of unicentric origin and spread peripherally, the tumor masses are not isolated but are connected with each other.
H and E, × 80

Fig. 114. Another case of superfical basal cell epithelioma.   ▷
H and E, × 100

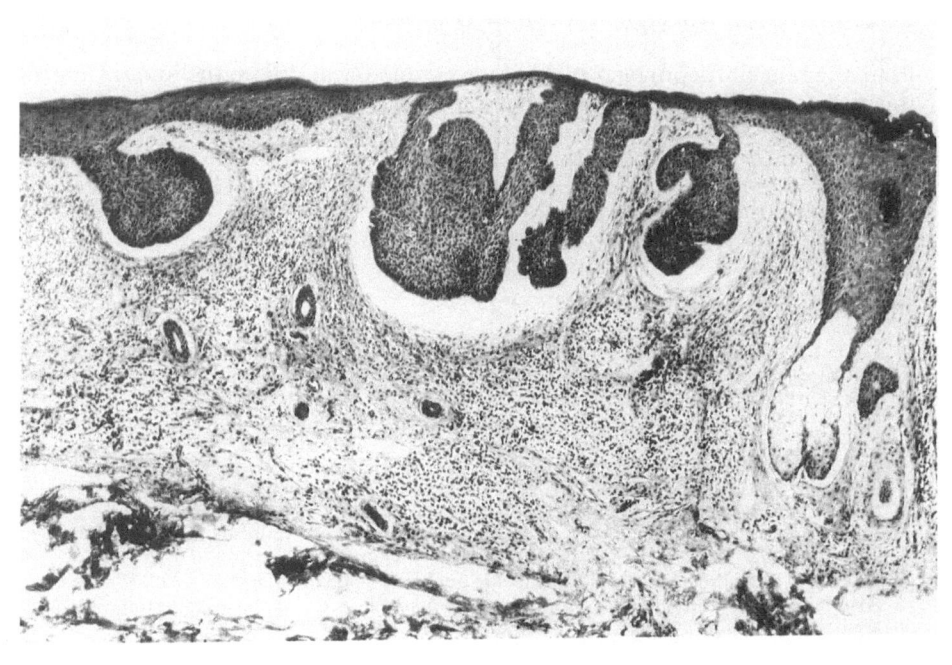

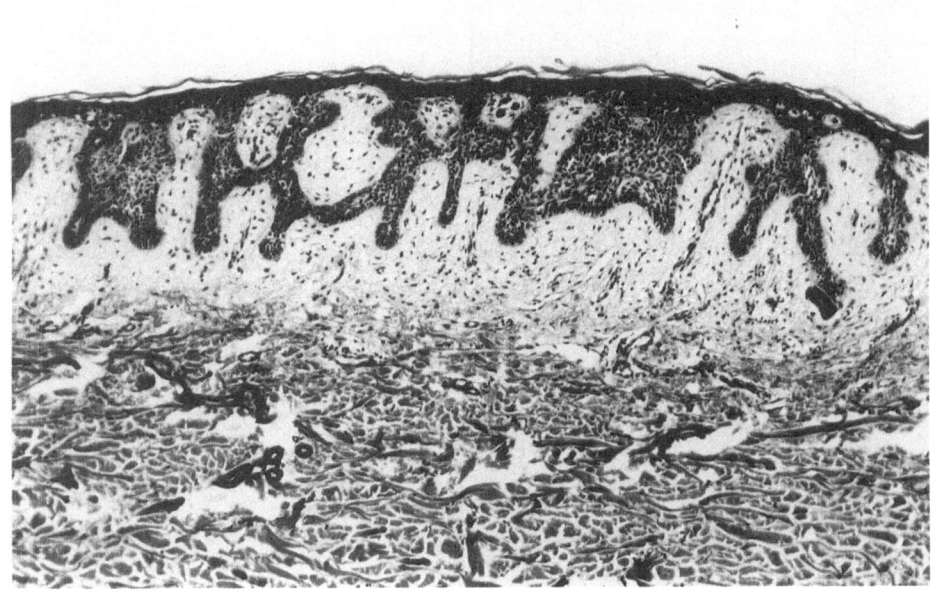

Premalignant fibroepithelial tumor (Pinkus)

Premalignant fibroepithelial tumor is a unique basal cell epithelioma. Clinically, this tumor is a fibromalike nodule and most commonly found in the lumbosacral region, but it may occur in the groin or elsewhere [7]. Grinspan and Abulafia divided it into three types—tumoral, papuloid, and en-plaque types [3]. Attention is now focused on a tendency of this tumor to arise in skin areas previously subjected to X-ray therapy [1,2,5,8–10].

REFERENCES

1 Colomb D, Bréchard JL, Gho A, Caux Y (1979) A propos de cinq nouveaux cas d'épithéliomas baso-cellulaires et de tumeurs fibro-épithéliales de Pinkus multiples du dos sur des zones ayant antérieurement été traitées par radiothérapie. Ann Dermatol Venereol 106: 875–822
2 Fawcett HA, Sanderson KV (1985) Fibroepitheliomata of Pinkus and basal cell carcinomata. Br J Dermatol 113 (Suppl 29): 54–55
3 Grinspan D, Abulafia J (1963) Tumor fibroepitelial de Pinkus. *Tumores fibroepiteliales premalignos de la piel (Pinkus)*. Arch Argent Dermatol 13: 23–44
4 Ishikawa K (1968) Premalignant fibroepithelial tumors of Pinkus. Jpn J Dermatol Ser B 78: 409–413
5 Marini D, Caccialanza M (1981) Influenza delle radiazioni ionizzanti sull'insorgenza di fibroepiteliomi di Pinkus. G Ital Dermatol Venereol 116: 483–488
6 Pinkus H (1953) Premalignant fibroepithelial tumors of skin. Arch Dermatol 67: 598–615
7 Posternak F, Civatte J (1976) Les tumeurs fibro-épithéliales de Pinkus à localisations extradorso-lombo-sacrées: A propos de 31 cas personnels. Ann Dermatol Venereol 103: 275–279
8 Rook A, Wilkinson DS, Ebling FJG (1979) Textbook of dermatology, 3rd edn. Blackwell, Oxford, p 2171
9 Sarkany I, Fountain RB, Evans CD, Morrison R, Szur L (1968) Multiple basal-cell epitheliomata following radiotherapy of the spine. Br J Dermatol 80: 90–96
10 Weitzner S (1972) Radiation-induced premalignant fibroepithelioma of the groin. Rocky Mt Med J 69 (no. 2): 49–51

Fig. 116. Small masses of basal cell epithelioma are arising from the lighter staining epithelial cord ▷ and have a budlike appearance.
H and E, × 320

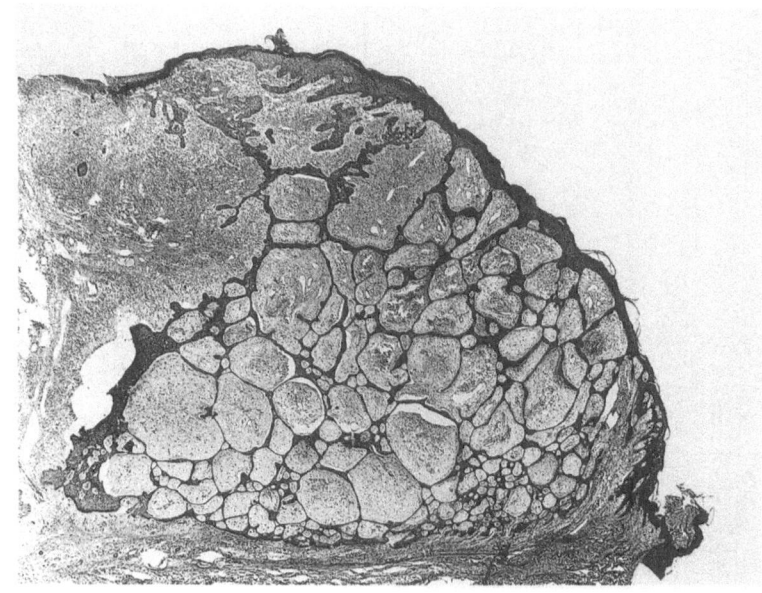

Fig. 115. An epithelial network, the cells of which are epidermoid in appearance, is embedded in an ample myxomatous stroma. The network is a histological manifestation of the tumor epithelium proliferating like the septa of a sponge.
H and E, ×15

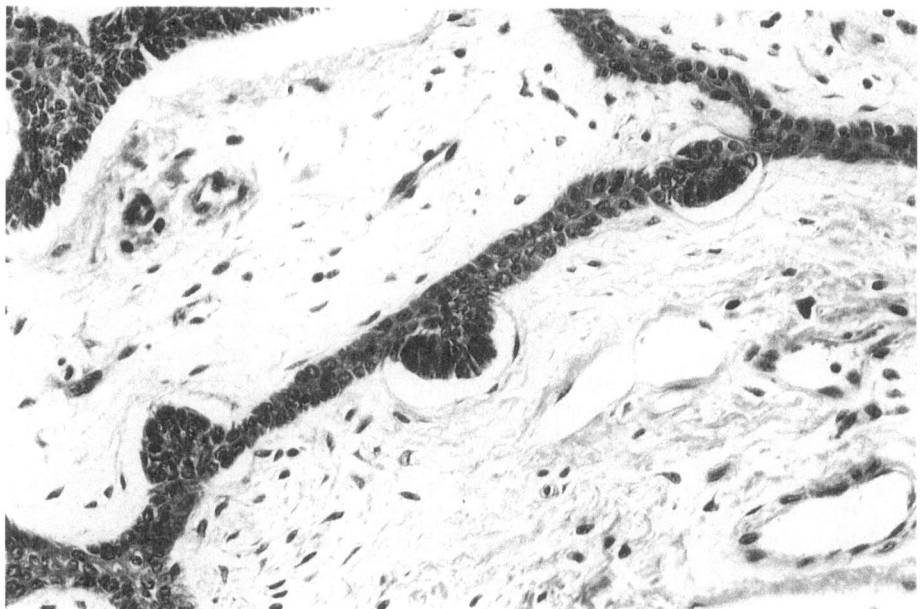

Subject Index